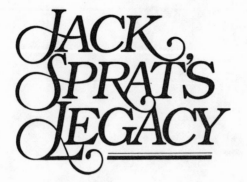

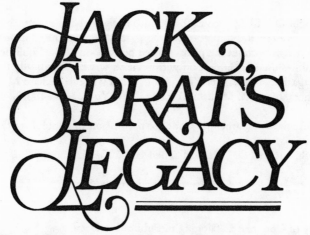

JACK SPRAT'S LEGACY

THE SCIENCE AND POLITICS OF FAT & CHOLESTEROL

PATRICIA HAUSMAN,
CENTER FOR SCIENCE IN THE PUBLIC INTEREST

FOREWORD BY RICHARD N. PODELL, M.D.
PREFACE BY MICHAEL F. JACOBSON, PH.D.

RICHARD MAREK PUBLISHERS
NEW YORK

Copyright © 1981 by Center for Science in the Public Interest
All rights reserved. No part of this book may be reproduced in any form or
by any means without the prior written permission of the Publisher, excepting
brief quotes used in connection with reviews written specifically for inclusion
in a magazine or newspaper. For information write to Richard Marek
Publishers, Inc., 200 Madison Avenue, New York, N.Y. 10016.

Grateful acknowledgment is made for permission to quote from the following
publications:
    Smith, Richard D. "Einstein: The Man." *The Washington Post*, March 11,
1979.
    Mayer, Jean (ed.). *U.S. Nutrition Policy in the Seventies*. W.H. Freeman and
Company, 1973.

Library of Congress Cataloging in Publication Data

Hausman, Patricia.
    Jack Sprat's legacy.

    Bibliography: p.
    Includes index.
    1. Nutritionally induced diseases.
2. Hyperlipemia—Complications and sequelae.
3. Hypercholesteremia—Complications and sequelae.
4. Food—Fat content. 5. Nutritionally induced
diseases—United States. 6. Nutrition policy—
United States. I. Title.
RA645.N87H38   616.1'071   80-26398
ISBN 0-399-90111-6

Design by Constance Sohodski

Printed in the United States of America

Acknowledgments

No words in this book are as easy to write as these, my thanks, to those who have contributed their time and talents to help me with this task.

Throughout the many months of research and writing, Joan Chernock provided invaluable administrative assistance. Michael Jacobson carefully read the manuscript and offered helpful suggestions. Miriam Daniel, Frances Collin, and Richard Podell also read drafts and offered constructive criticism. Eric Kilburn helped with research on pesticide residues in fat and early descriptions of heart disease. Anne Brown read thousands of pages of Federal Trade Commission testimony, summarizing it all onto a manageable stack of notecards. Leona Levine expertly typed the manuscript. Dave Pion helped with administrative work.

Mark Mayell deserves special thanks. He tabulated data on the fat content of foods and patiently worked with me designing and perfecting the Blood Cholesterol Scoreboard that appears in Chapter 7. Jan Zimmerman, Patricia Griffin, and Mike Leccese also helped manage the mountains of data. Bevi Chagnon of Art for People turned all the words and numbers into an eye-catching poster.

I would also like to acknowledge Dr. Thomas Kuhn, whose book, *The Structure of Scientific Revolutions,* has so much shaped my thinking, and Dr. Eleanor Williams, my professor at the University of Maryland. It was Dr. Williams who introduced me to the vast scientific literature on heart disease. She, more than anyone, turned my interest in nutrition into a passion. I am also indebted to more scientists, government officials, and industry representatives than I can name. Without their cooperation in granting interviews and providing information, writing this book would have been far more difficult.

Finally, a heartfelt thank-you to the friends who encouraged me so constantly: Robin Edelman, David Haber, Cece Cooney, and Bonnie Liebman. My deepest thanks go to my sister, Arlene Hausman, who made many personal sacrifices so that I might continue working on this book.

My editor, Joyce Engelson, helped me turn what can only be described as hamburger into what is hopefully ground round.

Patricia Hausman
Washington, D.C.
August 1980

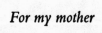
For my mother

Contents

Foreword

Jack Sprat's Legacy weaves together two tales of intellectual adventure. The first is the scientific search for the link between nutrition and heart disease. The second is the reaction of those for whom this search threatened cherished nutritional beliefs or economic interests. Together, these stories are essential background for people concerned about health—be it the public's or their own.

During the past forty years, physicians have identified several "risk factors" that predict an individual's chance of developing heart disease. The predictions are not perfect: a high probability of the disease is not the same as inevitability. Nevertheless, by analyzing a person's risk factors, physicians can estimate the individual's risk of heart disease—a risk that can vary as much as thirty times from one person to the next.

The most definite predictors of heart disease are a high blood cholesterol level, high blood pressure, cigarette smoking, and diabetes mellitus. Recently, scientists have identified some additional risk factors: sedentary life-style, Type A (overaggressive, time-pressured) behavior, and low levels of high-density lipoprotein.

11

Curiously, the public discussion of one of these risk factors—blood cholesterol—has lacked the dispassionate character one expects from scientific debate. Instead, intense emotion and even acrimony have prevailed. Among the other risk factors for heart disease, only cigarette smoking has stirred comparable passions, and I suspect for similar reasons. Both imply a need to change habits that are deeply imbedded in our culture. Both threaten important sources of economic livelihood.

Ms. Hausman writes as an advocate, but as an honest and meticulous one. She guides the reader along the various lines of evidence that form a persuasive case against the cholesterol-promoting eating style, which has long been a valued part of American culture. She recognizes that some uncertainty and grounds for continuing debate remain. However, she makes clear that the preponderance of evidence favors a change in diet for most Americans. She deals forcefully with the arguments often advanced to protect the dietary status quo.

Beyond this, and adding to our interest, Ms. Hausman describes the political and media battles waged by those with a deep emotional or financial stake in preserving current eating patterns. This is an exciting story and an important one. Its outcome will profoundly influence public understanding of the relationship between diet and coronary heart disease.

Richard N. Podell, M.D., M.P.H.
Director of Family Practice Education,
Overlook Hospital—Columbia University
College of Physicians and Surgeons
Summit, New Jersey

Dr. Podell is assistant clinical professor of medicine (family practice) at Columbia. He is board certified in internal medicine and family practice and holds a master's degree in public health. He serves as the chief medical consultant to the Health Systems Agency of New York City. He is a fellow of the American College of Physicians, American Academy of Family Physicians, and the American College of Preventive Medicine.

Preface
by Michael F. Jacobson, Ph.D., Executive Director, Center for Science in the Public Interest

A father of three dies suddenly of a heart attack at the age of forty-five. An elderly woman hobbles around feebly with her two canes, because of the arteriosclerosis in her legs. Gangrene forces the amputation of a business executive's leg. A sixty-year-old grandmother needs a hearing aid. An accomplished actress is felled in mid-career by cancer of the breast. A cerebral hemorrhage permanently cripples a physician on whom a small town relied.

These are the stories of all too many Americans. Every day, people who thought they were perfectly healthy suddenly discover that silently developing within them is a disease that ultimately leads to disability or death. While doctors have developed methods to prevent or cure most infectious diseases, they have found the chronic diseases much tougher to eradicate. The bacteria and other microbes that cause infectious diseases have no friends or allies to defend their interests and can be treated mercilessly as the health menaces they are. However, as

13

Patricia Hausman, a nutritionist who has worked for six years with great dedication at the Center for Science in the Public Interest (CSPI), documents in great detail and clarity in this book, some of the agents that cause degenerative diseases have powerful allies in the industrial world, academic community, and governmental bureaucracies, and are not so easily tackled.

Stroke, heart attack, and cancers of the colon and breast account for about one-half of all deaths in the United States. Countless medical researchers have devoted their lives to unraveling the causes of these diseases. Decades of research and literally thousands of scientific papers have identified some of the most important causes of many degenerative diseases. One major factor that stands out in study after study is the high fat content of the average diet. The old saying "We are digging our graves with our forks" was never more appropriate. This book is about how dietary fat and cholesterol, a related substance, speed the development of some of the most dreaded diseases and contribute to hundreds of thousands of deaths a year. These diseases include: coronary heart disease, peripheral arteriosclerosis, gangrene, hearing loss, cancers of the breast and colon, and cerebral hemorrhage.

Of all the problems that have been identified in foods in recent years—DDT, red dye No. 2, sugar, salt, cyclamate, saccharin, DES, excessive refinement, sodium nitrate, PCB, and PBB—fat is far and away the number-one problem. When people ask us at CSPI how they can improve their diets, we tell them that their highest priority should be to eat less fat, especially the saturated fat that is found in meat and dairy products, and cholesterol, which is abundant in eggs.

For some reason, health writers, with the notable exception of Nathan Pritikin and his colleagues, have sidestepped the number-one nutrition issue. Thus, we have had popular books about sugar *(Sweet and Dangerous)*, salt *(Killer Salt)*, vitamin and mineral deficiencies *(Nutrition Against Disease)*, and lack of roughage *(The Saccharine Disease)*, but no popular and authoritative treatise on fat. Perhaps, it is the enormous complexity of the fat/cholesterol

14

issue that has scared off the writers. Ms. Hausman's training as a nutritionist provided her with the necessary academic background to study and evaluate hundreds of scientific reports and mitigated whatever trepidation she might have had when she embarked on this two-and-one-half-year project. Ms. Hausman's intelligence and good judgment have enabled her to perform this job with a welcome degree of professionalism and intellectual honesty.

The first part of *Jack Sprat's Legacy* describes the mountain of scientific evidence that indicts the high-fat diet as a major killer, a killer of far more Americans than all our nation's wars combined. The evidence against fat is massive. The story begins with Russian studies on rabbits early in this century. Since then, experiments on numerous animal species, including monkeys, whose physiology and anatomy are remarkably similar to human beings, show that high-fat diets promote atherosclerosis and certain cancers. The most recent studies show that diets very low in fat can even reverse advanced atherosclerosis.

The conclusions drawn from animal studies are supported by several different types of human studies. Populations that consume a lot of saturated fat tend to have high rates of heart disease, while populations that eat little such fat tend to have low rates. Populations that eat large amounts of fat of *any* kind tend to have high rates of breast cancer and colon cancer. These epidemiological studies reveal associations between diseases and diet, but cannot *prove* a cause-and-effect relationship. For certain diseases, scientists can conduct tests on groups of human subjects to see if disease signs advance or recede when patients are exposed to various factors (drugs, diet, smoking, etc.). Such tests have shown that diets high in saturated fat and cholesterol promote heart disease. And as with the animal studies, new human studies are beginning to show that very low-fat diets can actually unclog arteries that were coated thickly with cholesterol plaque.

As a practical matter, it is impossible to prove with absolute certainty that a particular factor, like diet, causes a chronic, degenerative disease. To do this would require a study in which large numbers of identical twins were separated at birth and raised identically for the the rest of their lives in every respect except, for instance, their fat and cholesterol intakes, which would be adjusted by the researchers. Obviously, a study of this sort would last several decades and cost millions of dollars. But even this kind of study could be questioned, because it might prove impossible to raise the separated twins in an identical fashion. Regrettably, the opponents of a low-fat diet are demanding that essentially impossible studies be done before agreeing that the government should encourage the general public to alter its diet. The limited, but vocal, opposition to dietary changes helps make this subject—and this book—such a fascinating one.

The second part of this book (chapters 9 to 11) focuses on the "fat lobby": the meat, dairy, and egg industries, and their academic and political allies. These three industries, which together provide about 60 percent of the food we eat, have been vigorously fighting efforts to change certain aspects of the American diet. Not too long ago, the nutritional worth of meat, dairy products, and eggs was unquestioned. After all, these foods were loaded with vitamins, minerals, and protein. But the discovery by scientists that meat, dairy products, and eggs were contributing to diseases that have reached epidemic proportions has put these multibillion-dollar industries on the public health "hit list." Patricia Hausman provides example after example of how farm interests and food processors have opposed policies and programs that would improve the public's health, but endanger the industries' profits.

Over the years, the "fat lobby" has not only influenced our nation's food and nutrition policies, it has *determined* those policies. The meat, dairy, and egg industries have enormous influence in the House and Senate agriculture committees. Rare is the legislator who will resist the pleas of farmers, if they make up a significant number of voters in his or her district. How a legislator will vote on an issue is almost foreordained when unorganized consumers with a diffuse interest in the issue are opposed by phalanxes of lawyers and scientists representing an industry that is aggressively defending a narrow, strongly felt economic interest.

Recently, the meat, dairy, and egg industries have begun using advertising in the mass media and professional journals to influence the general public and nutritionists. Madison Avenue jingles ("The incredible, edible egg"), billboards ("Milk is for Everyone"), and print ads ("Beef: Nutrition You Can Sink Your Teeth Into") sing the praises of the foods and seek to blunt our interest in the saturated fat and cholesterol that so readily clog our arteries.

In virtually every school district in the country, the minds of two generations of children have been fed the self-serving pap served up in generous portions by the National Dairy Council, a nonprofit arm of the dairy industry. Needless to say, the dairy group extols the virtues of milk, cream, cheese, and ice cream, making only the barest, briefest, rarest mentions of the health problems caused by diets high in fat and cholesterol. Other industries also provide nutrition education materials to schools, though not on such a grand scale.

Frequently, when industry amasses its troops on one side of an issue, forces dedicated to consumers' interests coalesce in response. The two most serious health problems caused by high-fat diets are heart disease and cancer. One would expect that the American Heart Association and the American Cancer Society would be at the forefront of the battle. Sad to say, that is not the case.

The American Heart Association has sponsored a great deal of excellent research and did lead the battle against high-fat diets back in the 1960s. On the basis of growing scientific evidence, it advised the public to cut down on saturated fat and cholesterol. Almost single-handedly, the AHA made saturated fat and cholesterol an issue, and its activities met with some success. However, the hotter the battle became, the more reluctant the Heart Association behaved. Instead of providing outspoken public leadership, Heart Association officials retreated into scientific meetings and laboratories. The Heart Association, with its tens of millions of dollars of income, could be fighting for labeling that would highlight the fat content of foods, for reduced fat levels in hot dogs, and for major nutrition education campaigns in schools and on radio and television. The Heart Association has done none of these things.

The American Cancer Society has been, if anything, less progressive than the heart group. During the 1970s scientists discovered that lifelong diets high in fat and cholesterol appeared to increase the risk of cancers of the breast and colon. Animal studies showing that high-fat diets were linked to cancer had been performed as long ago as the 1930s. Also, pesticides and other potentially cancer-causing toxic chemicals tend to accumulate in the fatty tissue of livestock and fish. Either of these factors should have caused the American Cancer Society, the nation's largest voluntary health organization, to swing into action. The Cancer Society could have supported tighter restrictions on pesticides, more nutrition education, and other measures that would have helped reduce the risk of cancer. In fact, an alliance between the Cancer Society and Heart Association might have been an unbeatable combination. The hundreds of local chapters and thousands of volunteers might have been able to generate political pressure dwarfing that produced by the meat, dairy, and egg interests. Unfortunately, the Cancer Society has done virtually nothing.

Despite the massive amount of scientific evidence linking fat to heart disease, a relative handful of researchers has created in many minds the illusion that great controversy surrounds this "theory." Perhaps the press, too, deserves some criticism here, because for the sake of a "story" all too many reporters eagerly seize upon a dissenting view without questioning its validity or the credibility of the dissenter. Though the arguments made by critics of the diet-heart relationship often sound reasonable, closer examination usually reveals that the critics are misinterpreting the evidence, intentionally ignoring a multitude of studies that do not support their argument, or demanding impossible-to-obtain evi-

18

dence, evidence they cannot produce for their own favorite notions.

While the underlying motivation of the critics of dietary change is impossible for an outsider to fathom, many of these purportedly unbiased researchers have egregious conflicts of interest. For instance, in June 1980, a committee of the National Academy of Sciences issued a report defending the current fatty diet. The main authors of the report were professors who had for many years received grants from or were paid consultants to the National Dairy Council, National Livestock and Meat Board, American Egg Board, Kraft Foods, General Foods, and other industries whose profits depend on Americans' pathogenic diet. One such professor was quoted in the press as being surprised that people thought that the $250,000 he has received as a consultant to the egg and other industries would cloud his objectivity regarding the nutritional value of eggs. These same professors, perhaps with the aid of their corporate friends, have ensconced themselves in numerous other governmental and professional committees. Meanwhile, the great majority of more independent academics has been extremely reticent to participate in the politicking inherent in battling for more enlightened nutrition policies. The public's health has suffered immeasurably because of that reticence on the one hand, and the eager involvement, often whetted by money, of industry-oriented scientists on the other hand.

The U.S. Department of Agriculture (USDA) has been the federal agency responsible for nutrition education. Until 1977, the department's official position was "all food is good food." USDA's nutritionists, pamphlets, and books found something good to say about everything from hot dogs to candy bars. Every food had a place in the diet. The only diet-related diseases that were officially recognized were scurvy, beri-beri, and other vitamin-deficiency diseases. The diseases that were caused in part by eating too much of certain foods produced by any of USDA's important farm constituencies—such as the meat, dairy, and sugar industries—were conveniently ignored.

Since 1977, the federal government has changed its position on nutrition at a pace that must have caused vertigo in untold numbers of career bureaucrats accustomed to snail-paced changes and in corporate executives accustomed to having things their own way. Largely because the industry-oriented Nixon-Ford appointees at the departments of Agriculture and Health, Education, and Welfare were replaced by President Jimmy Carter's more consumer-oriented appointees, the government began providing sensible nutrition advice to the public and progressive leadership to health professionals. Now the official policy on nutrition is to eat less fat, cholesterol, refined sugar, and salt. And this is what the pamphlets, TV spots, and books are beginning to say.

The people who deserve the most credit for this remarkable turnaround are, first, citizens in every corner of the country who have been writing letters to politicians, starting food co-ops, organizing natural foods fairs, and doing a hundred other things to educate the public and our "leaders"; and, secondly, a handful of Washington officials: Senator George McGovern, who headed the Senate Select Committee on Nutrition and Human Needs; Secretary of Health, Education, and Welfare Joseph Califano, who released the Surgeon General's Report on Health Promotion and Disease Prevention, which encouraged sensible nutritional practices; and Secretary of Agriculture Bob Bergland and Assistant Secretary Carol Foreman, who converted their department from an industry fiefdom to an agency that would listen to consumers. Two Harvard nutrition professors, Mark Hegsted, who later became director of USDA's human nutrition research, and Jean Mayer, now president of Tufts University, deserve special mention for providing an academic stamp of approval for the new nutrition policies that challenged the farm lobby and food processors.

The government's about-face on nutrition did not occur without great opposition, opposition that has not ceased to be active. It will be interesting to see if the growing constituency for nutrition—both in and out of government—can hold its own in the 1980s. The challenge facing nutrition advocates in the coming decade will be to convert an official policy that exists only on a sheet of paper into real programs that actually bring more healthful food to the table. The election in 1980 of a Republican administration, which has close ties to agribusiness, and a conservative Republican senate, coupled with the defeat of Senator McGovern, indicates that the challenge will be met only with the most vigorous and persistent activism by health advocates.

While this book is primarily about the health problems that a high-fat diet causes, its topic is also a microcosm of many contemporary health controversies. Should diseases be prevented, even if this means urging life-style or behavioral changes on some people who would never have gotten the disease? To what extent should the government be in the business of advising people how they should eat or otherwise live their lives? Who will represent the interests of the unrepresented citizens, especially the poor and uneducated? Does industry support for academicians undermine or co-opt a traditional bastion of objectivity? Does industry have excessive influence on national policies? Clearly, questions such as these are not even limited to health policies, but apply to most of the other dilemmas that face our society.

Whether these vital health and other issues are resolved in a way that is beneficial to the general public interest or to narrower, vested interests will depend largely on the degree of involvement of people as active citizens. Policy arenas, such as Congress, are like city parks. The amount of crime, fear, and skullduggery goes down as the number of citizens present goes up. Active public involvement and scrutiny is one of the greatest protective devices known. *Jack Sprat's Legacy* is like a breath of fresh air compared to most other books about nutrition, because it transcends nutrition and explores the underlying causes of diseases that have their roots more in economics and cultural patterns than in lack of scientific knowledge. If we, citizens working together, can beat back the economic, industrial, and political forces that are literally killing us by dietary means, we will also see the way to protecting and preserving the public's best interests on other fronts. The underlying message of this book is that to maximize our health it is necessary, but not sufficient, to change our personal eating habits. We must also dedicate ourselves to improving broad national policies that have great impact on all our lives.

Washington, D.C.
November 1980

JACK SPRAT'S LEGACY

1

Deprogramming
the Basic Four

When mighty roast beef was the Englishman's food
It ennobled our hearts and enriched our blood
Our soldiers were brave and our courtiers good
Oh! the roast beef of old England!
       Richard Leveridge
       British vocalist, songwriter, and composer
       1670–1758

Richard Leveridge was a songwriter, but he might have been a nutritionist. From its beginnings, the science of nutrition has given high marks to meat, or to any food that contains generous amounts of protein, vitamins, and minerals. Though Leveridge is gone, his philosophy is with us to this day—epitomized, perhaps, in the recent words of Nebraska Senator Carl Curtis:

Now, of course, the most nutritious food you can eat is meat. It makes for stronger bodies. In the whole history of the world, whenever a meat-eating race has gone to war against a non-meat-eating race, the meat-eaters won. It produces superior people. We have the books of history.

Were Leveridge alive today, he, like Curtis, would find company among the old school of nutrition—the school that emphasizes protein, vitamins, and minerals and little else—save

25

weight control. Nutrients have been the theme of nutrition research for almost two centuries. Nineteenth-century scientists noted the need for protein, carbohydrate, fat, and minerals. Turn-of-the-century researchers discovered another class of nutrients: the vitamins. Around 1913, two University of Wisconsin researchers, Dr. Elmer McCollum and Marguerite Davis, discovered a substance in milk fat and egg yolk that was essential to the growth of laboratory rats. They had found the first vitamin: vitamin A.

At the same time that McCollum and Davis found an essential nutrient in milk fat and egg yolk, Russian scientists discovered that rabbits fed these two foods developed atherosclerosis, a hardening of the arteries. Atherosclerosis is the underlying cause of most heart attacks and strokes, the major causes, respectively, of death and disability in the United States.

The findings of the Russian scientists, though, went virtually unnoticed by nutritionists. Nutrition science took the other road, studying the beneficial elements in food, with little consideration to the possibilities of harm. Following the discovery of vitamin A, nutrition scientists became captive to nutrients. Research focused on finding nutrients, synthesizing them, estimating daily needs, and measuring the amounts in the diets of people around the globe. To the nutrition scientist, the only harmful substance in food was one that interfered with the body's use of a nutrient. And meat, milk products, and eggs—all rich sources of nutrients—became the nutritionist's all-star foods. Sugar, with no nutrients, was branded the worst of the lot.

It was not surprising that science took the nutrient road, ignoring research linking the fat of meat, milk, and eggs with atherosclerosis. At the turn of the century, a heart attack or stroke was a luxury that too few lived long enough to experience; infectious diseases and malnutrition took much younger lives. Tens of thousands of Americans developed pellagra, a disease caused by too little niacin in the diet; vitamin D deficiency crippled—and killed—young children. Even Elmer McCollum, the discoverer of vitamin A, had suffered scurvy during his first year of life. He might have died had his mother not unwittingly fed him apple scrapings one day. Noticing that he seemed to like them, she continued to do so. The vitamin C in the apple peel was enough to cure McCollum's disease, though his mother never knew why the symptoms disappeared.

The choice to follow the nutrient road was also consistent with other social goals. At the turn of the century, much of the population earned its living by farming. Nutrition research was not seen simply as an investment in human health, but also as a means of helping farmers. To produce healthy livestock at a low cost, farmers needed a better understanding of the animals' nutrient needs.

The dedication to the nutrient needs of livestock was so great that when Elmer McCollum first requested funds to study the needs of rats, the dean of the University of Wisconsin College of Agriculture was enraged. McCollum recalled the conversation well:

> Dean Russell listened with ill-concealed irritation. When I stopped talking he had the answer on the tip of his tongue. It was no. We were to experiment with economically valuable animals. The rat was a pest to farmers. If it ever got noised about that we were using federal and state funds to feed rats we should be in disgrace and could never live it down.

The dean, however, relented and agreed to permit the rat colony after an influential scientist popular with the dairy farmers intervened on McCollum's behalf. In the long run, the dean's fears proved unfounded, for McCollum's work with the rats uncovered an essential vitamin in milk fat. After the discovery, wrote McCollum, "he [Dean Russell] was delighted, for he well knew with what enthusiasm such an announcement would be received by dairy farmers everywhere." Having grown up on a farm himself, McCollum was happy to be of help to farmers. No doubt many of his colleagues had been raised on a farm as well and were dedicated to its needs.

Farmers and nutrition scientists became fast friends. Farmers donated money for nutrition research and for public education about nutrition. In return, nutrition scientists untangled mysteries of nutrient needs, enabling farmers to improve their herds and tout the nutritional attributes of their products. Farming and nutrition science were almost viewed as a single entity; some universities even delegated the teaching of nutrition to departments of dairy and animal science.

There was a third party in the scenario: the government. The government was eager to participate in nutrition activities, which seemed to yield benefits for both farmers and consumers. It was the federal government that translated knowledge developed in the laboratory into advice for the general public. By World War II, nutrition research had uncovered so many essential nutrients that teaching the public about the sources of each one became impractical. Home economists at the U.S. Department of Agriculture (USDA) simplified the detailed knowledge of nutrients into a food guide called the Basic Seven. Citizens were taught to choose foods from each of the seven groups. The Basic Seven had a place for every food; it was built on the premise that every food had one or more nutrients to contribute to the diet.

In 1956, USDA nutritionists pared the seven food groups down to four. The Basic Four Food Groups—dairy, meat, fruits and vegetables, and breads and cereals—has been the nutrition education gospel ever since. Like its predecessor, the Basic Four gave no demerits; it merely stressed eating a variety of foods. The farmers and the food industry liked the approach. In fact, one farm-sponsored group, the National Dairy Council, was so enthusiastic about nutrition education a la the Basic Four that the government took the backseat, allowing the Dairy Council to become the country's major provider of nutrition education materials.

The Basic Four seemed to be serving the nation well. By the mid-fifties, when the four food group plan was developed, nutrient deficiencies that had plagued Americans during earlier decades had been wiped out. American nutritionists were sum-

Nutrient Deficiencies: A Steady Decline

Registered Deaths in the U.S. from:	1917	1927	1937	1947	1957	1967	1977
Pellagra (niacin deficiency)	3,666	5,418	3,258	728	76	13	0
Rickets, osteomalacia (vitamin D deficiency)	566	475	252	53	21	5	9
Scurvy (vitamin C deficiency)	94	42	27	22	4	1	3
Beri-beri (thiamin deficiency)	15	8	21	49	40	8	8
All causes	1.1 million	1.2 million	1.4 million	1.4 million	1.6 million	1.9 million	1.9 million

29

moned to developing nations to do for those countries what they had done for their own. In some of the developing world, U.S. nutritionists encountered high rates of deficiency diseases that they had hardly ever seen in their own country—notably protein-calorie malnutrition that took the lives of thousands of preschool children. Knowing that those who ate meat, milk, and eggs rarely developed the disease sold nutritionists all the more on the wisdom of the Basic Four.

For the science of nutrition, the first half of the twentieth century had been like a 1930s musical. Everyone was happy with the fruits of nutrition research. There was something for everyone: the farmer, the researcher, the U.S. citizen, and the child in the developing world.

But the happy days didn't last forever. There was still that matter of the rabbits developing atherosclerosis when fed a diet rich in the fat of meat, milk, and eggs. Most nutritionists had ignored the findings, but medical researchers had taken up where the Russian scientists left off. They took the Russians' findings far past rabbit experiments, to studies with animals more similar to humans and then to studies with humans. They compared disease rates among countries. By the 1960s they could not help but conclude that the Basic Four was not serving us well enough. American men, despite their diet rich in protein, vitamins, and minerals, were about six times as likely to die of heart attacks as Japanese men. Rates of certain cancers also differed dramatically between the two countries; colon and breast cancers were five times as common in the United States.

Researchers realized that pollution, smoking, and hectic life-styles were not the likely explanation; the United States and Japan had all three in common. Study after study implicated diet as an important explanation for the differences. The most outstanding difference between the Japanese and American diets was the fat content; Americans were eating two to four times as much fat as the Japanese. The message was that some of the nutritionist's most revered foods were not so flawless after all. Despite their nutrient value, egg yolk, and certain meat and dairy products are

30

high in fat or cholesterol, a fatlike substance also linked to heart disease.

The conclusions of the heart and cancer researchers transformed the field of nutrition from a 1930s musical to a documentary of war. As late as 1977, many nutritionists would not accept proposals to lower the fat content of the American diet. "The American diet is better today than ever before and is one of the best, if not *the* best, in the world today," said Dr. Gilbert Leveille, chairman of the Department of Food Science and Nutrition at Michigan State University.

At the St. Louis University School of Medicine Dr. Robert Olson argued, "It is ironic that beef, whose consumption in countries all over the world has been associated with the best overall health statistics, is now under attack. . . . It is felt by zealots attacking beef that eggs and whole milk, which are equally nutritious foods, should be abandoned because they contribute unnecessarily and disproportionately to our present burden of chronic disease."

And Dr. Fred Kummerow, a professor of food chemistry at the University of Illinois, insisted that the American diet is "the most economical, most nutritious diet ever available to man."

Other nutritionists tried to make the problem of heart disease fit into the nutrient view, proposing that nutrient deficiencies, not excesses of fat and cholesterol, were responsible for high rates of heart disease. They tried to blame heart disease on deficiencies of vitamins, on imbalances of minerals, and, of course, on the nutritionists' longtime villain—sugar. But the amount of evidence incriminating these was small compared to the volumes of evidence already accumulated against fat and cholesterol.

Still others tried not to deny the relationship between high-fat foods and heart disease but to ignore it. Nutrition textbooks kept the benefits of fat in the spotlight, giving little attention to the heart disease research. "The discussion of the relationship of dietary fat and atherosclerosis in an elementary text can be legitimately questioned," wrote Dr. Helen Guthrie in the 1975 edition of *Introductory Nutrition,* one of the most widely used

31

university nutrition textbooks. Nutritionists still considered it more legitimate to discuss deficiency diseases that were now all but nonexistent in the United States. (*Introductory Nutrition* devoted an equivocating page and a half of its 500 pages to the subject of diet and heart disease.) Future nutritionists were trained to believe that little research had been done and that few conclusions could be made.

But if nutritionists had listened to their colleagues in heart research and said, "Yes, of course," to the evidence against meat fat, milk fat, and egg yolk, it would have been a first in science history. "Science often suppresses fundamental novelties because they are necessarily subversive of its basic commitments," wrote science historian Dr. Thomas Kuhn in *The Structure of Scientific Revolutions*. The heart researchers' conclusions couldn't have been a bigger affront to the basic commitment of nutritionists: the Basic Four. It was a challenge not just to commonly accepted notions about the most nutritious foods, but also to the most fundamental assumption in nutrition: *that nutrition is the study of the beneficial elements in food*. Accepting the heart researchers' conclusions meant a drastic redefinition of nutrition: to include not just the pluses in food, but also the minuses. It was a change that scientists trained in the nutrient view of food would not readily accept—just as centuries before, scientists who regarded the earth as the center of the universe steadfastly rejected Copernicus's conclusions that the earth, in fact, revolved around the sun.

Innovators in any field had to survive the inevitable opposition of established professional attitudes, but in nutrition, defenders of the American diet were not the scholars alone. The farmers, the food industry, and the government had been fond supporters of the strictly positive approach to nutrition. As heart scientists proposed that Americans cut back on fatty meat and dairy products, farm groups reacted with disbelief, despair, and defensiveness.

Medical research had done the same thing to tobacco farmers. They had grown tobacco long before science had anything to say about it, only later to hear it stand accused as a major cause of disease and death. "These [tobacco] farmers are not immoral at all," John Pinney, director of the government's Office of Smoking and Health, told a reporter in 1980. "They are doing something their forebears have done for 250 years. It is a tragedy that they are caught up in one of the great public health problems of our time."

It was apparent that meat, dairy, and egg farmers might become act two of the tragedy. Science had not only not criticized them when they began to raise their animals, but had actually praised them. Now, science was pulling the rug out from under them. The meat, dairy, and egg groups followed in the footsteps of the tobacco farmers and looked to their longtime ally, the government, for assurances that their interests would be upheld.

Finding a friend in the government was not difficult. The U.S. Department of Agriculture, the de facto protector of the American farmer for more than half a century, was happy to stick its head in the sand on the issue of fat, cholesterol, and heart disease. In 1976, USDA Assistant Secretary Richard Feltner revealed that his agency was still adhering to the strictly positive view of nutrition—despite two decades of warnings about fat and cholesterol. "Essentially all foods marketed provide food energy and/or at least a small amount of one or more nutrients and are therefore recognized by ARS [USDA's Agricultural Research Service] as nutritious," Feltner told congressmen.

Even agencies not directly devoted to the needs of farmers were careful to stay out of the fracas. The bureaucracy at the Department of Health, Education and Welfare—including the Food and Drug Administration, the National Institutes of Health, and the HEW coordinating office—was tight-lipped on the subject of fat and cholesterol. Agency officials would cite the "controversial" nature of the proposed diet changes as their defense, but under tough questioning it turned out that even these agencies felt a loyalty to agriculture that influenced their decision to keep quiet.

In 1978, New York Congressman James Scheuer demanded an explanation for HEW's silence. With the Food and Drug Administration's top nutritionist, Dr. Alan Forbes, before him Scheuer asked about the advice to cut back on fat, cholesterol, salt, and sugar.

"Sir, there is a great deal of scientific support for this general approach," replied Forbes.

"Do you have a political problem in sending out that message?" the congressman asked.

"I presume we probably would," conceded Forbes.

Later in the hearing, Dr. Michael McGinnis, HEW's deputy assistant secretary for health, told Congressman Scheuer that HEW was still hesitant to give advice about fat and cholesterol to the public.

"Is that a political problem or a scientific problem?" the astute congressman asked.

"Well, I suspect it is a bit of both," replied McGinnis.

At the National Institutes of Health (NIH), HEW's scientific conscience, it turned out that even the definition of "scientific proof" was influenced by political considerations. Dr. Robert Levy, director of NIH's National Heart, Lung, and Blood Institute (NHLBI) conceded that the evidence required for an NHLBI policy on fat and cholesterol must be stronger than for issues that don't cause problems for economic interests. "I would guess that since there are these [meat, dairy, and egg] interest groups one is going to need harder scientific data to confront them. . . . One can't deny that as long as there's a group outside with commercial interests, it's going to be harder to achieve change," said Levy in 1978.

Though Congressman Scheuer seemed to believe that federal agencies should put the public's health in front of political considerations, Congress itself had not always set a good example. In 1978, members of the House Agriculture Committee, conceding to pressure from the meat and egg industries, defeated the National Consumer Nutrition Information Act, a bill that would have increased federal funds for nutrition education. Congress also passed promotion programs designed to increase the consumption of meat and eggs. Laws initiated to protect the farmers' interests remained on the lawbooks even after it became clear that the provisions violated the health interests of the nation.

Efforts to spread the word about eating less fat and cholesterol faced still another obstacle: a country sated with seemingly endless, often contradictory warnings about what not to eat. Advocates of lower-fat diets recommended more low-fat dairy products, lean meat, poultry and fish, and fruits, vegetables, and grains. But newspapers warned about pesticide residues on the fruits and vegetables . . . toxic chemicals in the fish . . . carcinogens in mushrooms, apple cider, and tea. Weight-loss mythology had convinced almost everyone that bread and potatoes were fattening. Adding high-fat foods to the "eat less" list made it seem like there was nothing left to eat—nor to drink. Even the water reportedly had carcinogens. And when toxic chemicals were found in the last sacred food—mother's milk—the conclusion was obvious: Life is nothing but Russian roulette and trying to beat the odds in such an arbitrary game is a waste of time. Even some of the scientists who discovered the risks in food or drink admitted that they, too, were sick of hazard chic and were wondering if trying to heed the warnings was worth it.

But the new school emerging in the nutrition field was content with neither the outdated principles of the Basic Four nor with the argument that avoiding hazards had become a full-time job, too cumbersome to handle. Actually, the new school in no way rejected the notion that protein, vitamins, and minerals are vital to health. *Rather, it added a new dimension: that a good diet is one that limits fat and cholesterol at the same time that it meets nutrient needs.* The salt and sugar content of the American diet also became a concern, as did the effects of refining grains. And to those who argued that the hazard list had become unmanageable, the new school proposed that a pecking order be established among the hazards so that the most serious could be avoided while the rare dangers be given lower priority.

The new school found a friend in Congress: the Senate Select Committee on Nutrition and Human Needs. The committee, chaired by Senator George McGovern, had been convened in

1968 to investigate hunger and malnutrition among the nation's poor. But half a decade into its work, the committee realized that America's affluent also suffered from nutrition problems. Its work expanded to include hearings about the role of diet in heart disease, cancer, and other health problems. By 1977, the committee—like nutrition's new school—was convinced that the high fat content of the American diet was one of the most serious hazards facing the country. It put out a report that said just that: advising Americans to eat less fat and cholesterol, as well as less salt and sugar. The report was called *Dietary Goals for the United States*—but as far as the farmers and many nutritionists were concerned, it might well have been called *Future Shock*.

Almost overnight, farm groups demanded withdrawal of the report. Mail flooded the committee's offices. Political pressure forced the senators to hold hearings where farm interests took issue with the recommendations. Not surprisingly, scholars accustomed to viewing nutrient deficiencies as the only diet-related diseases were quick to challenge the report's advice. At the University of Wisconsin, nutrition professor Dr. Alfred Harper protested, "To what extent are the diseases for which the dietary goals have been described nutritional diseases? Not one of them is a nutritional deficiency disease. They are all diseases of complex and not clearly understood etiology. There is great disagreement over how important nutrition is as a factor in their development."

Dr. Cortez Enloe, publisher of *Nutrition Today* magazine, concurred. "One thing—and little else—is clear after reading the dietary goals that Senator McGovern and his staff want the nation to pursue. Politicians make poor scientists and scientists make poor politicians."

And suddenly, nutritionists and farm groups who had welcomed that government invention called the Basic Four were complaining that "the government should not tell people what to eat." The National Dairy Council, which had spent decades happily informing children that the government advises them to drink three to four glasses of milk per day, angrily retorted that it was inappropriate for the government to set levels for the desirable amount of fat in the diet. It was obvious that the Dairy

Council wanted nutritional advice from the government only if "eat more," not "eat less" was the credo.

But an impressive group of scientists defended the *Dietary Goals*. "This is a long overdue set of recommendations vital to the health of the United States," wrote Dr. William Kannel, director of the government's Framingham Heart Study. "The goals stated are widely supported by those interested in the prevention of cardiovascular disease, despite the impression created by a vocal minority that receives too much attention from the press and the medical journals."

"Generally speaking, I think this report constitutes a major breakthrough," wrote another heart expert, Duke University's Dr. Siegfried Heyden. "My only concern is that not enough publicity has been given to the Senate report when it was published in February of 1977. After you have received all additional comments that you have requested, you should launch a major press campaign in order to bring the content of the Senate report to the attention of every American."

And to those who argued that "the government should not tell people what to eat," Dr. Henry Blackburn, heart researcher at the University of Minnesota, gave this reply:

Inalienable as are personal freedoms and rights of choice, it is surely considered socially ethical to promote a personal practice and a public policy that discourage self-destruction and encourage health! Values, likes, cravings, and aversions are strongly culturally determined. A sound public health policy needs to clarify those values, to present and encourage more healthy tastes. A free people have nothing to fear from personal knowledge and awareness of risk, from a better discrimination between destructive and healthful life-styles, or from an atmosphere conducive to positive health and well-being in contrast to self-indulgence and overconsumption.

To say the least, the Senate committee—which had become a subcommittee of the Senate Agriculture Committee soon after releasing the *Dietary Goals* report—heard every argument in the book. Despite months of intense pressure from farm interests and like-minded scientists, the arguments of the scientists supporting the *Dietary Goals* were too convincing for the senators to ignore. In the end, the nutrition subcommittee refused to retract the report—or even to make substantial changes. "We don't particularly enjoy making recommendations that get us into political trouble back home," McGovern explained to egg farmers. "These findings don't come to us easily. They are findings that the committee has shared because we thought they were in the best interests of the health of the American people. We want to do what we can to ease the economic impact of the recommendations on any industry. We can't do that at the expense of what we believe is the health of the American public."

The USDA and HEW were compelled to take a look at the evidence against fat and cholesterol—evidence apparently so strong that senators vulnerable to political pressure would not bow to the protests of American agriculture. The agencies formed their own committees to evaluate the *Dietary Goals*. After two more years of government silence, the Surgeon General issued a report urging Americans to eat less fat and cholesterol. The same year, the National Cancer Institute put its imprimatur on the "less fat" advice. Finally, in 1980, even the USDA joined with the Department of Health and Human Services (formerly HEW) in issuing "dietary guidelines" that followed the recommendations in the *Dietary Goals*. Americans, said all three reports, should eat more low-fat dairy products, lean meat, poultry, fish, and vegetable foods. Fats, oils, fatty meats, high-fat dairy products and egg yolks, they said, should be reduced. Even a few food companies nodded in agreement.

Some dissenting nutritionists bit the bullet and stopped campaigning against the new advice. A few continued to beat the protest drums loudly. In 1980, the Food and Nutrition Board of the National Academy of Sciences, a group composed mostly of nutrient specialists, made a last-ditch effort to save the Basic Four. In a brief report entitled *Toward Healthful Diets* the board

38

challenged the government's advice on fat and cholesterol. But board members succeeded mostly at making fools of themselves. Major newspapers criticized the report's content and the board's one-sided membership of scientists who had long opposed recommendations for dietary change. Most important, the Surgeon General and the government agencies stood firm.

Farmers continued to believe that they had been unjustly vilified. "I suggest that the committee who wrote *Dietary Goals* must have been influenced by the unsaturated fats lobby, the vegetarians, the food faddists, and the people who think we should feed the Third World," an enraged pork producer wrote to Senator Charles Percy. Little did he realize, the farmers had not lost a war to another special interest group, but to an idea whose time had come.

2

Too Much of a Good Thing

Adelle Davis probably brought more life to the subject of nutrition than all of her critics combined. While the standard nutrition textbook bored its students with dry, easily forgotten descriptions of the many nutrients and their functions, Davis fascinated her readers with memorable stories of people who were transformed from hopeless cripples to Olympic champs by simple changes in their diets.

For every nutrient, Davis had a heartwarming, but not necessarily believable, story. In *Let's Eat Right to Keep Fit,* she told of an eighteen-month-old boy plagued with severe eczema almost since birth. She recalled feeding him six or eight tablespoons of soybean oil, which he gobbled voraciously. She advised his parents to feed him several tablespoons of the oil every hour if he wanted it. Only three days later, she reported, the eczema had disappeared, and the parents were so grateful that Davis commented, "If there is one man in the world willing to die for me, it is probably this boy's father." Fat must be amazing stuff.

Davis attributed the child's dazzling improvement to linoleic acid, a constituent of fat abundant in most vegetable oils. Linoleic acid is essential for growth and healthy skin, and because the body cannot make its own supply, the diet must provide it.

Science has other kind words for fat: it carries vitamins A, D, E, and K and helps the body absorb them. Fat contributes to satiety, the feeling that one's had enough to eat. Fat also supplies calories in a more concentrated form than protein or carbohydrates. Gram for gram, fat has more than twice the calories of protein or carbohydrate. These concentrated calories cause problems for many of us, but are vital for infants. Infants grow very rapidly during the first year of life, and the calorie needs of this time cannot be met by low-fat diets. The recommendations in this book are not suitable for children under one year of age.

Obviously, fat plays a crucial role in nutrition, making unique contributions to our health. However, as amazing as its life-sustaining properties is the smallness of our need for it. To absorb vitamins properly, about 10 percent of the calories in the diet need to come from fat. To prevent the scaling skin and poor growth that Adelle Davis described the fat called linoleic acid must represent about 1 to 2 percent of the calories in the diet—much less than the six tablespoons she fed the young child. Diets with only 10 percent of the calories from fat usually meet the linoleic acid requirement; keeping the fat content of the diet this low requires a fish and vegetable diet and these foods contain ample amounts of linoleic acid. The good health of cultures eating a low-fat diet confirms that the need for fat is small. American visitors to Japan, where the traditional fish and rice diet averages only 10 percent of its calories from fat, have not returned with tales of a scaly-skinned people suffering from stunted growth.

While a diet as low in fat as traditional Japanese cooking adequately meets our fat requirements, the American diet averages 40 percent of its calories from fat—too much of a good thing. Nutrition textbooks tend to be long on the benefits of fat and short on the hazards, but most make at least a passing comment in favor of eating less fat.

To cut down on fat, one has to know where it's coming from.

It does come from foods thought of as "grease": butter, margarine, salad oils, and frying fats. But these are only part of the story. Fat in meat, chicken, and fish—sometimes hidden from view—as well as the fat in milk, cheese, and other dairy products supply as much of our fat as the "grease." The rest of our fat comes in small doses from nuts, chocolate, avocadoes and coconut (all rich in fat) and the tiny amounts in other fruits, vegetables, grains, and beans.

Sources of Fat in the American Diet★

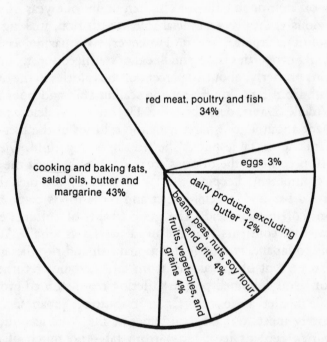

red meat. poultry and fish
34%

eggs 3%

cooking and baking fats,
salad oils, butter and
margarine 43%

dairy products, excluding
butter 12%

beans, peas, nuts, soy flour,
and grits 4%

fruits, vegetables, and
grains 4%

Nutritionists use several methods to measure fat in foods, and two of these are useful to consumers. The first method—listing

★"Nutrient Content of the National Food Supply," R. Marston, L. Page. *National Food Review,* pp. 28–33, U.S. Department of Agriculture, December 1978.

the grams of fat in a serving of food—is commonly used by companies that provide nutrition information on their food labels. The grams-per-serving method allows easy comparisons among foods as long as serving-sizes are equal. Three ounces of cooked hamburger has 17 grams of fat; three ounces of cooked chicken meat, 6 grams. Breyer's vanilla yogurt has 7 grams of fat per carton, while Dannon's has 3 grams. The lower fat choices are obvious. However, when serving-sizes designated by manufacturers differ among brands, easy comparisons are no longer possible. And lowering your daily fat intake by counting grams of fat usually isn't practical. To watch your fat consumption by the grams method you need a scale to weigh servings of solid food; a measuring cup for liquids, a food diary, a table of food composition, a calculator, and an unlimited supply of patience.

Another problem with the grams method is that we eat by calories, not by grams of food. Our need for food reflects the calories we burn, not a demand for 800 grams of food per day. Comparing grams of fat among foods with very different calorie values is truly like comparing apples and oranges. Two foods may each have 10 grams of fat in a serving, but if one has 500 calories and the other 100 calories, the fat content is hardly the same.

The easiest way to understand this concept is to imagine a diet containing only one food. A diet containing 1,500 calories per day that contains only the food with 10 grams of fat per *500* calories would have only 30 grams of fat. On the other hand, a 1,500-calorie diet based only on a food that contains 10 grams of fat per *100* calories would have 150 grams of fat—quite a difference. Ideally, the measurement of fat in food should reflect both fat and calorie content. This is the purpose of another method of measuring fat: the percentage-of-calories method.

The percent of calories from fat represents the portion of a food's calories contributed by fat. If fat provides 40 percent of a food's calories, the remaining 60 percent come from protein, carbohydrate, or alcohol. This method simplifies the fat and calorie content into one value that remains the same regardless of serving size. Apples and oranges may now be compared; the percentage method tells whether 200 calories of apples has more or less fat than 200 calories of oranges. (The difference between the two fruits is negligible, but enormous when fatty meat is compared to lean meat.)

Emphasizing the foods where fat provides a low or moderate percentage of the calories is an easier way to lower your fat intake than counting every gram. Nonetheless, this method is not perfect, and there are instances where the grams method is better. Fat provides half the calories in both mustard and whole milk, but whole milk drinkers probably consume more fat from milk in a day than from several months' worth of mustard. Olives derive about 90 percent of their calories from fat, which seems like a great deal, but olives have so few calories and are eaten in such small quantity that their fat is not important in most diets. Evaluating foods by the percentage-of-calories method is a poor technique for condiments, low-calorie foods, and anything eaten in small amounts. Grams per serving is useful in these cases. Knowing that a teaspoon of mustard has 0.3 grams of fat and two green olives 1 gram tells you that their fat content is pretty irrelevant (unless you eat them by the jar).

Both the grams and the percentage method will be used throughout this book. For perspective, a food can be considered low in fat if fat provides fewer than 30 percent of its calories; from 30 to 50 percent, the fat content is moderate; above that, high. In cases where grams of fat per serving best describes fat content, less than 5 grams means a low-fat food, six to 10 grams represents a moderate fat content; and more than 10, a high fat content.

The method of measuring fat that rarely will be used in this book is the percentage of fat by weight. Agriculture scientists began using this method decades ago, and it is still a practical technique for their purposes. Unfortunately, it has been abused as a clever way of deceiving consumers about the fat content of food.

When expressed as a percentage of a food's weight, the fat content of most foods will sound deceptively low. Whole milk, for instance, contains only 3 to 3.7 percent fat by weight, simply because milk, like most foods, contains large amounts of water. By weight, whole milk is 87 percent water. But fat supplies half the calories in whole milk; a glass has 8 grams of fat. What sounds like a small amount by the percentage weight method is actually quite a bit.

Even the fat content of solid foods sounds low when expressed as a percentage of the food's weight. Half a hot dog's weight is water; its fat content amounts to 30 percent by weight. But from the standpoint of calories, a hot dog is mostly fat, and Oscar Mayer would rather you not know. In its pamphlet, *Myths and Facts about Meat Products,* the company uses that 30 percent figure to fool you about the fat content of a hot dog:

Myth: Sausage products, including weiners and cold cuts, are "fatty."

Fact: The federal government has established a maximum 30 percent fat content for some processed meats, including weiners and bologna . . .

The fact is that fat supplies 80 percent of the calories in a hot dog—certainly enough to justify the "fatty" label.

Not only the amount of fat in the American diet, but also the kind of fat causes problems. Fats fall into three categories, based on the amount of hydrogen that can be added to them. A saturated fat has all the hydrogen that it can hold. Monounsaturated fats can hold two additional hydrogen atoms, while polyunsaturated fats can accommodate at least four additional hydrogen atoms. To the chemist, this is just the beginning; scientists have isolated 34 different saturated fats, 26 monounsaturated fats, and 18 polyunsaturates. However, only a handful of these predominate in food. Within the categories the differences are not very important; one polyunsaturate affects blood cholesterol levels the same as another. Some saturated fats affect the body differently than others, but all foods rich in saturated fat contain enough of the type linked to heart disease that fine distinctions about the various kinds of saturated fat aren't necessary. Ditto for the mono-saturates, as only one type is common.

Calculating the Percentage of Calories from Fat

1. Multiply the number of grams of fat per serving by 9.
2. Divide the result by the number of calories per serving.
3. Multiply the result by 100.

Example: Low-fat cottage cheese (2 percent milk fat by weight)

Serving size:	½ cup
Calories per serving:	101
Protein:	16 grams
Carbohydrate:	4 grams
Fat:	2 grams

Step One: 2 grams fat (per serving) × 9 calories (per gram of fat) = 18 calories from fat per serving.

Step Two: 18 calories from fat per serving ÷ 101 calories per serving = 0.18.

Step Three: 0.18 × 100 = *18 percent of calories from fat.*

All foods contain a mixture of the three types of fat. For simplicity, nutritionists often refer to a food's fat as "saturated" even though some mono-unsaturated and polyunsaturated fat is present. This shorthand is based on the relative amounts of the three kinds of fat. *Saturated* is a fair label for a fat in which saturated fats supply one-third or more of the fat. *Polyunsaturated* aptly describes vegetable oils and fish fats that contain less than 15 percent of their fat in the saturated form and at least one-third polyunsaturated fat. The term *mono-unsaturated* applies to fats that also have less than 15 percent of their fat in saturated form, but less than one-third polyunsaturated fat. The following chart shows where common fats fall when classified in this manner.

Shorthand Classification of Some Common Fats

Saturated	Mono-unsaturated	Polyunsaturated
Beef, pork, and lamb fats	Olive oil	Corn oil
Milk fat	Peanut oil	Safflower oil
Coconut oil	Some margarines	Sesame seed oil
Palm oil	Some vegetable shortenings	Soybean oil
Some industrial shortenings		Sunflower seed oil
		Many fish fats
		Some margarines

The last item on the fat agenda is the cholesterol in food. Unlike fat, cholesterol has no calories, and it belongs to a different class of chemicals. Nevertheless, scientists often refer to cholesterol as a fat because it has similar effects on the body. Cholesterol in blood and cholesterol in food are the same substance; scientists use the jargon "dietary cholesterol" when speaking of the cholesterol in food and "plasma cholesterol" or "serum cholesterol" when referring to the same substance in the blood. For most uses, the simpler terms food cholesterol and blood cholesterol suffice to distinguish between the two.

Only animal foods contain cholesterol in amounts worth talking about. Egg yolk is the most common high-cholesterol food, and organ meats also have large amounts. Shrimp is moderately high. Red meats, poultry, and fish have less cholesterol than these others, but sometimes have much more saturated fat. Both saturated fat and food cholesterol influence blood cholesterol levels, though of the two, saturated fat is more important.

Sources of Cholesterol in the American Diet*

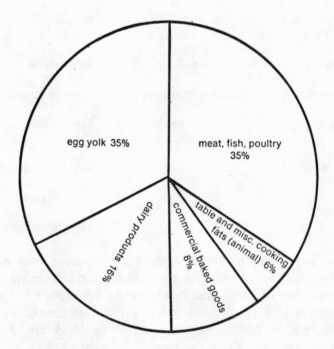

*Based on: Stamler, J., in *Reprints from Ischaemic Heart Disease*, FADL-Forlag, 1977.

Too Much of a Good Thing

Cholesterol in the American diet averages 400 to 500 milligrams (mg) per day. For decades, nutritionists never gave much thought to the cholesterol, nor to the 80 grams of fat that usually accompany it. But today, research makes clear that this diet has had its price: the world's second highest rate of coronary heart disease.

3

All That Human
Hearts Endure

Cowpox was once nothing more than a cattle disease, but
Edward Jenner turned it into a blessing for man. Jenner was an
English physician who found that inoculating people with bits of
material from cowpox lesions gave them immunity from smallpox. Millions of people have been vaccinated since his 1796
discovery, so successfully that the once-epidemic smallpox has
been eradicated from every corner of the globe. Only laboratory
samples of the smallpox virus and a debt of gratitude to Edward
Jenner remain.

Jenner made other contributions to medicine, but none as
celebrated as his smallpox vaccine. Another of his fascinating
discoveries was made as he conducted an autopsy. In his
memoirs, he gave these details:

> My knife struck something so hard and gritty as to notch it. I
> well remember looking up at the ceiling, which was old and
> crumbling, conceiving that some plaster had fallen down.

But on further scrutiny, the real cause appeared: the coronaries [coronary arteries] were become bony canals.

Other scientists of his day came across the same curiosity. In 1705, physiologist William Cowper observed an artery that "very much resembled a bit of the stem of a tobacco pipe, its sides were so thick, and its bore consequently much lessened." Cowper called the thick deposits "ossifications and petrifactions." Jean Baptiste Sénac described an artery that was "hard as a bone, like branches of coral."

Jenner, Cowper, and Sénac were all taking about the same thing: arteriosclerosis, or hardening of the arteries. In the most common form of arteriosclerosis, fatty substances, notably cholesterol, accumulate in the artery walls. This type is known as atherosclerosis, and the fatty deposits are called plaques.

Atherosclerosis progresses slowly throughout life. Most cardiologists believe that it begins in childhood, with harmless "fatty streaks" in the arteries (Figure 1). The fatty streaks gradually fill with cholesterol and other fatty material. As the process advances the arteries become hard and inelastic. The plaques protruding from the artery wall interfere with the flow of blood. Often, the plaques affect the coronary arteries that supply the heart with blood, and the inadequate blood supply to the heart muscle causes angina pectoris (chest pains). But just as often, people with severe atherosclerosis in their coronary arteries have no symptoms at all. Eventually, though, a blood clot may form along a plaque or a plaque itself may grow so large that the flow of blood to the heart is blocked. Suddenly, a seemingly healthy person becomes a victim of a heart attack. If the same process occurs in the brain arteries, the victim has a stroke.

Heart attacks and strokes are everyday occurrences in the United States. With all the numbers in, the nation's heart attack toll comes to 1.25 million per year, of which 650,000 attacks are fatal. In the case of stroke, 200,000 victims become death statistics each year. At the National Heart, Lung, and Blood Institute, director Robert Levy estimates that 84 percent of these 850,000 deaths involve atherosclerosis in some way.

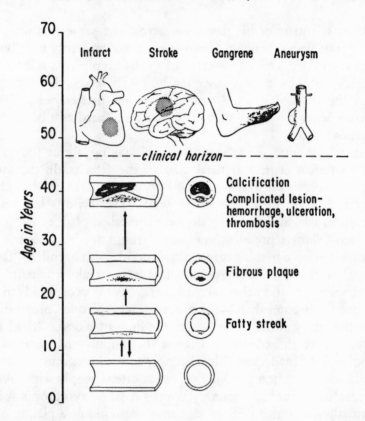

Figure 1: The progression of atherosclerosis, from early to advanced stages.*

Atherosclerosis affects our "hearts and minds" most commonly, but other parts of the body sometimes succumb to its ill effects. The body's main artery, the aorta, as well as arteries in the neck, arms, and legs can be affected. Pain after eating or exertion is common when these arteries are clogged, and doctors call the

*From *Atherosclerosis and Its Origin,* H.C. McGill, J.C. Geer, J.P. Strong. 1963. Reprinted courtesy of Academic Press and M. Sandler and G.H. Bourne, eds.

condition peripheral vascular disease. Unchecked peripheral disease can lead to gangrene, the destruction of body tissues caused by an inadequate supply of blood. A few studies also link atherosclerosis to loss of hearing during later life.

Despite a wealth of knowledge about atherosclerosis, folklore on the subject abounds. Popular fiction holds that people like Edward Jenner made diseases caused by atherosclerosis unavoidable by controlling infectious diseases and allowing us to live longer lives. There is a grain of truth to the idea. Atherosclerosis rarely takes its toll before middle age, and if smallpox killed most of us before then, only a few would have a chance at heart disease. Control of infectious diseases makes degenerative diseases more likely, but not inevitable. Atherosclerosis is not as inevitably linked to aging as the annual accumulation of rings around a tree.

Nothing speaks to the potential for preventing atherosclerosis as well as the International Atherosclerosis Project, a worldwide study of heart disease and stroke conducted from 1963 to 1965. After examining the arteries of 20,000 autopsied people in sixteen cities, scientists concluded that where a person lived greatly influenced the severity of plaques in his arteries. The average middle-aged white man in New Orleans, for example, had more than twice as much advanced atherosclerosis in his coronary arteries as his Mexican neighbor of the same age (Figure 2). Black men in New Orleans, aged forty-five to fifty-four, averaged three times as much severe atherosclerosis as black men of the same age residing in Puerto Rico or Brazil.

Atherosclerosis showed the same variation in the brain arteries as in the coronary arteries. Men in Norway, for instance, had more severe brain plaques than men of the same age in Guatemala. The degree of atherosclerosis also proved to be critical. Everyone had some plaques, but the study found that complications arose only after large amounts had accumulated. The differences in severity of plaques from country to country explained the differences in rates of heart disease and stroke. The conclusion was obvious: Plaque deposits varied so much among countries that aging alone could not be solely responsible for the

Distribution of Coronary Atherosclerosis★

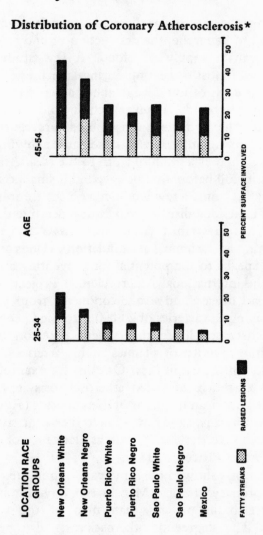

Figure 2: Variation in atherosclerosis among men in different locations. Black bars represent percentages of the coronary arteries affected by advanced plaques. The dotted bars represent fatty streaks.

★From *The Geographic Pathology of Atherosclerosis,* Henry McGill, ed., 1968. Reprinted courtesy of the U.S.-Canadian Division of the International Academy of Pathology.

problem. It seemed that life-style must play a major role in atherosclerosis.

At the turn of the century, long before the International Atherosclerosis Project was on the drawing board, a scientist named Sir William Osler also noticed that atherosclerosis didn't strike blindly, but in a pattern. The rich, he noted, succumbed to the complications of atherosclerosis far more often than the poor. He reasoned that the differences in diet might explain the phenomenon; the rich ate meats and other fatty foods, while the poor ate mostly low-fat grains. Osler proposed that atherosclerosis was the "Nemesis through which Nature exacts retributive justice for the violation of her laws."

It was only a few years later that Russian scientists produced evidence that Osler was on the right track. In 1908, the Russian scientist Ignatowski found that rabbits fed meat, milk, or eggs developed atherosclerosis while those fed a vegetable diet did not. Ignatowski thought the animal protein was responsible, but a few years later, another Russian, Anitschov, showed that the fat and cholesterol were the culprits.

Scientists were cautious not to draw final conclusions from the rabbit experiments. The rabbit's plaques didn't resemble human's very well, and the search continued for a more suitable test animal. Chickens came next, and though they developed atherosclerosis if fed a diet high in fat and cholesterol, their plaques also didn't match human's closely enough. Studies with dogs and rats, then monkeys and swine followed. All developed atherosclerosis on a high-cholesterol diet, though the dog was resistant unless fed huge amounts. Not surprisingly, the plaques of human's closest relative, the monkey, matched human atherosclerosis very well.

Diets like the one Americans consume have produced grim results in the monkey's arteries. At the University of Chicago, Dr. Robert Wissler and his colleagues fed rhesus monkeys a typical American diet. A second group of monkeys received a modified American diet lower in fat, cholesterol, and calories, but not drastically different from our usual menu. The first group of monkeys liked the food, but paid a price: six times as much atherosclerosis as the monkeys on the lower-fat meal plan. Plaques in the coronary arteries were four times as severe in the monkeys eating the typical American diet.

Scientists have not only produced severe atherosclerosis by feeding monkeys the American diet; they've successfully un-clogged arteries by switching animals from high-fat, high-cholesterol diets to lower-fat fare. At the University of Iowa, Dr. Mark Armstrong and his co-workers fed a diet rich in egg yolk fat and cholesterol to monkeys and found that more than half their coronary arteries were blocked by plaques. After switching some animals to a diet low in fat (or high in polyunsaturated fat) for a year and a half, only one-third as much atherosclerosis was found.

No one will ever be sure that people respond to their diet exactly the same way that monkeys do. But one thing is certain: the experiments done with monkeys can't be done with people. People don't live in cages where everything they eat and all aspects of their life-styles can be controlled. Moreover, you can't kill them when you decide it's time to look at their arteries. You have to wait for a natural death, and that means an experiment that would last for decades.

This state of affairs is nothing new in science; the perfect proof is often impossible to obtain. Hopefully, no one would deliber-ately expose people to a suspected cancer agent to see what happens. Instead, cancer testing relies on animal experiments and epidemiology, the study of factors associated with disease. When both animal and epidemiological studies implicate something as a cause of cancer, the researchers are usually convinced.

Epidemiological studies of atherosclerosis show the same results as the animal studies. Worldwide, every population that has a high rate of heart disease eats a diet rich in saturated fat and cholesterol. In an international study, Dr. Ancel Keys and his colleagues chemically analyzed the food eaten by men in seven countries. They found that the heart disease rates in each area closely matched the amount of saturated fat in the men's diets. Fat consumption was closely related to severity of plaques in the International Atherosclerosis Project as well. White subjects in New Orleans had the most severe plaques, and the Norwegians in Oslo were second. Fat consumption was highest in these two cities. (No distinctions about the kind of fat were possible, but high-fat diets are usually high in saturated fat.)

Atherosclerosis wasn't built into the genes of Norwegians and Americans. Studies of migrating populations show major changes in heart disease rates as people move from country to country. The Japanese are a case in point: when Japanese eating a low-fat diet migrated to Hawaii and tripled their fat intake, they also increased their risk of serious atherosclerosis. Dr. Ancel Keys and his colleagues found that Hawaiian Japanese aged fifty to sixty-nine were twice as likely to have severe atherosclerosis as men of the same age still living in Japan.

The experience of the Japanese migrants confirms the findings of the International Atherosclerosis Project—that environment or life-style, not heredity, influences atherosclerosis the most. No doubt family history and genetics play some role in an individual's risk of heart disease, but the great differences in heart disease rates among populations clearly result more from life-style than from genetic factors.

Whether changes in life-style can unclog human arteries as successfully as monkey arteries is a major issue, and the answer may not be a simple yes or no. The prospects may depend on how far the plaques have progressed and what steps are taken to unclog them. But there is reason for optimism—heart disease rates dropped during food-scarce (and fat-scarce) wartime, and scientists believe that regression of atherosclerosis may have occurred. Cancer patients, who often lose weight rapidly, have shown shrinking plaques. And in closely monitored studies using a new technique called angiography, scientists have documented plaque reduction in patients who lowered their blood cholesterol and blood triglyceride levels. Triglycerides are a type of fat found in the blood.

Angiography is similar to X-rays, and heart surgeons use it to study the condition of patients' arteries before surgery. Of the various kinds of evidence favoring the possibility of plaque reversal, angiograms are held in highest esteem. The angiograms can be very precise, high-quality evidence if done properly. And experiments showing reduction of plaques in patients who lower their blood cholesterol levels support the link between diet and heart disease. Blood cholesterol levels are considered the "mechanism," that is, the process by which saturated fat and cholesterol influence atherosclerosis.

Nothing makes scientists happier than finding a physiological explanation to account for associations between life-style and disease rates. A correlation between a habit and a disease doesn't necessarily mean that the habit causes the disease. Everyone has heard of nonsense correlations; the number of liquor stores in U.S. cities correlates closely with the number of ministers. Does this mean that ministers inspire drinking? No one would argue that it does, but many try to deny the link between saturated fat and heart disease by pointing to nonsense correlations such as this. But for heart disease, the correlation with saturated fat and cholesterol looks like anything but nonsense; there are other kinds of experiments—and a mechanism—to support it. Pieced together, the evidence paints a cause-and-effect relationship involving three steps:

Step One: Saturated fat and cholesterol in the diet increase the blood cholesterol level.

Step Two: The higher the blood cholesterol, the greater the rate of plaque formation in the arteries.

Step Three: The more severe the plaques in the arteries, the greater the risk of heart disease, stroke, and other complications of atherosclerosis.

The validity of the link between diet and heart disease is obvious when the evidence is evaluated in this step-by-step format. Human studies show that cholesterol and the type of fat in the diet do influence the level of cholesterol in the blood. Saturated fat raises the blood cholesterol level (Figure 3); mono-unsaturated fats have little effect. The polyunsaturated fats lower the blood cholesterol level. Saturated fat is the prime influence; a gram of it raises blood cholesterol twice as much as an equal amount of polyunsaturated fat lowers it. Food cholesterol also raises blood cholesterol (Figure 3) but has less effect than saturated fat.

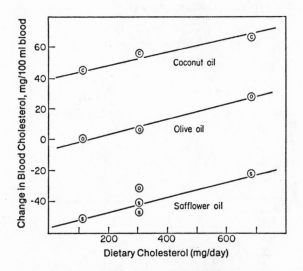

Figure 3: The effect of different fats and food cholesterol on blood cholesterol levels.* With only 100 mg food cholesterol in the diet, a diet in which coconut oil (a saturated fat) replaced the usual fat in the American diet raised blood cholesterol levels an average 46 mg. At the same low level of food cholesterol, olive oil (a mono-unsaturated fat) had a neutral effect, causing only a 1 mg increase in blood cholesterol. The safflower oil (a polyunsaturated fat) lowered blood cholesterol levels an average 52 mg at this low level of food cholesterol. As food cholesterol was increased to 300 mg and 600 mg per day (small circles), cholesterol levels increased, regardless of the type of fat in the diet.

*Graph courtesy of R. B. McGandy and D. M. Hegsted. Reprinted with permission from *The Role of Fats in Human Nutrition*. A. J. Vergroesen, ed. Copyright by Academic Press, Ltd. (London), 1975.

Evidence that the amount of cholesterol in the blood affects the severity of plaque comes from both animal and human studies. Scientists have had no trouble demonstrating this relationship in animal experiments (Figure 4). The International Atherosclerosis Project provided human evidence to support the animal findings; the average blood cholesterol level in each city closely matched the severity of the plaques. More direct evidence in humans comes from a study with terminally ill patients. Scientists injected radioactive cholesterol into their blood, and this cholesterol was found in their plaques when they died.

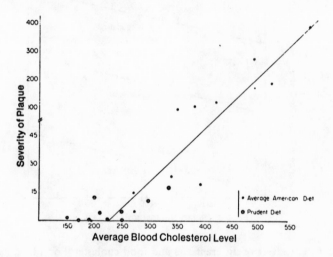

Figure 4: The relationship between the average cholesterol level during a two-year period and the severity of plaques in two groups of monkeys.* Monkeys fed a diet containing moderate amounts of fat and cholesterol (large circles) generally had lower blood cholesterol levels and mild plaque. Monkeys fed a typical American diet, high in fat and cholesterol (small circles), had higher blood cholesterol levels and more severe plaques in the aorta.

*Graph courtesy of Dr. Robert Wissler and the American Health Foundation conference on optimal blood lipids. Published in *Preventive Medicine*, November 1979. Reprinted with permission of Academic Press.

Angiography has also provided evidence that blood cholesterol influences the buildup of plaque. One study found blood cholesterol levels 20 to 40 percent higher in patients with severe plaque than in people with less serious atherosclerosis. The experience of people affected with a rare genetic disorder causing extremely high cholesterol levels also supports the relation between blood cholesterol and plaque. People with this condition can have cholesterol levels three times higher than the average level. Their atherosclerosis is early and severe, and complications often take their lives in young adulthood.

Almost everyone agrees with step three: that the plaques built up in the arteries contribute to heart disease and stroke. In the International Atherosclerosis Project, victims of heart disease averaged three times as much advanced atherosclerosis as those who died in accidents or from diseases unrelated to atherosclerosis.

Research showing a strong relation between blood cholesterol levels and the chances of heart disease strengthens the evidence against diet further still. Scientists believe the relation is a continuous one, with risk of heart disease rising as the cholesterol level increases. (Blood cholesterol is measured in milligrams per 100 milliliters of blood, but it's common practice to express cholesterol levels simply as a number, without the descriptive "milligrams per 100 ml.") Below a level of 180, a man's risk of heart disease is small, but the chances start to rise slowly with increasing levels. Beyond a level of 250, the risk jumps sharply (Figure 5). Cholesterol levels are also a risk factor for stroke in men under the age of sixty. However, high blood pressure is the most important risk factor for stroke, and if a high cholesterol level is also present, the risk intensifies. The relationship between blood cholesterol and heart disease has not been extensively studied in women, but the information available does show that a woman's risk increases as the blood cholesterol rises. The difference is that at the same level of blood cholesterol, a woman has a lower risk than a man, simply because she is female.

Rates of First Heart Attack per 1,000 of Male Population

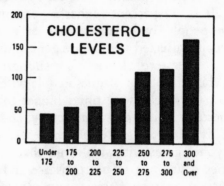

Figure 5: The risk of first heart attack, per 1,000 men, at various levels of blood cholesterol.*

"There is no controversy that [blood] cholesterol is a risk factor," says Dr. Robert Levy, director of the National Heart, Lung, and Blood Institute. After the word *controversy,* he backtracks to make himself clear. "There is no *intelligent* controversy," he says the second time around. However, recent research focusing on where the cholesterol is carried in the blood has led others to believe that the cholesterol level itself (and therefore the diet) no longer indicates the risk of heart disease.

Cholesterol in the blood is carried by fat-protein complexes called lipoproteins. The low-density lipoproteins, LDL for short, carry most of the cholesterol. The LDL have long been regarded as the culprit in atherosclerosis. High-density lipoproteins, or HDL, carry smaller amounts of cholesterol, and other lipoproteins have still smaller quantities. Recent research shows that, of the various blood fats, cholesterol carried by the HDL is the most important heart disease risk factor among people older than fifty-five. In this case, it's a low level that carries the greatest risk, unlike the case with the total blood cholesterol or LDL-cho-

*Graph courtesy of National Heart, Lung, and Blood Institute, Framingham Heart Study.

62

lesterol level where a high level signals danger. These new findings have been touted as evidence clearing diet of a role in heart disease, as scientists believe that diet does not have major effects on HDL.

Scientist-writer Richard Passwater, for instance, interpreted the HDL research in this way:

> Telling yourself how much [total] blood cholesterol you have is like telling yourself something about the size of shoe you wear. It has no meaning at all. . . . I think the worst form of food faddism is someone who fears the use of eggs, meat, and dairy products because [he fears] they will give him heart disease. I think cholesterolphobia is an unneeded, unfounded fear of eating good foods.

A writer for *Apartment Life* magazine was just as optimistic:

> A balanced diet—one that includes a wide variety of foods— is coming back as rule number one for good nutrition. And if you follow it, you really don't have to get too hung up about no-no foods, including [fatty foods] . . . which have been on the blacklist for 30 years. . . . Some misinterpreted statistics many years ago caused a lot of doctors to jump on the cholesterol bandwagon. . . . Recent studies just haven't produced any firm evidence that cholesterol in the diet is the cause of common kinds of heart disease. It seems if you've got a lot of HDL, it doesn't matter how high your total blood cholesterol levels go, or (within reason) what you eat.

And our center's mailbag bulged with letters urging us to come out of the Dark Ages and realize that the findings on HDL had cleared meat fat, butter, and egg yolk from any role in heart disease. A member from Albany wrote:

> The saturated vs. unsaturated fat theory is also pretty hoary and has been poked full of holes. Even Framingham [a well-

known heart disease study] is backing off on dietary cholesterol since HDLs came to the fore.

From upstate New York came another chiding letter about our
views on saturated fat and cholesterol:

Most of what I have read of late on this subject seems to
indicate that this is really not as important as was once
thought and, in fact, may be unimportant. The Cholesterol
Theory has been promoted by the medical establishment for
a long time with complete disregard for any facts or findings
to the contrary.

And from New York City, these words:

I'd like to be involved in your organization but your views
on cholesterol are archaic.

HDL is important. But diet is important too.

The HDL findings have obscured the important fact that LDL
levels of cholesterol and total cholesterol levels are still related to
risk of heart disease. At every age studied, either the LDL level or
the total blood cholesterol level is a significant risk factor for a
heart attack. As far as science knows, saturated fat and cholesterol
affect mostly the cholesterol carried by the LDL. In other words,
blood fats influenced by diet remain important factors in heart
disease. A high level of HDL-cholesterol isn't good enough if the
cholesterol carried by LDL is also high, and examples from recent
research show why. When results from several studies were
combined, scientists found that men with high HDL-cholesterol
levels (above 53) had a heart attack rate of 85 per 1,000 men if
their LDL-cholesterol levels fell between 140 and 179. Men with
the same high levels of HDL but with LDL-cholesterol levels of
180 or more had 130 heart attacks per 1,000 men—a 50 percent
greater risk!

Knowing both the HDL and LDL levels of cholesterol in your

blood allows the most precise measure of your risk of heart disease. Nonetheless, the total level of cholesterol, which combines the amount carried by the LDL, HDL, and other fat-protein complexes, is usually a good measure of risk. The total blood cholesterol and the LDL-cholesterol are strongly related. If total cholesterol is too high, chances are very good that the fat-sensitive LDL-cholesterol is also too high. The chances that a high cholesterol level will result from a high level of the beneficial HDL are small. At the University of Minnesota, researchers found that only ten percent of men and women with high cholesterol levels fell into the lucky category where the explanation was a generous level of HDL.

No blood cholesterol level is guaranteed to prevent heart attacks. The statisticians simply tell us that the odds of suffering a heart attack worsen as the cholesterol level rises; they don't draw a line between safe and unsafe. But people are accustomed to neat cutoff points dividing "normal" from "abnormal," and statisticians often define all values except the uppermost (or lowest) 5 percent as "normal." It isn't unusual to hear all blood cholesterol levels below 300 labeled "normal," because only 5 percent of the U.S. population has higher levels. But "normal" in the statistical sense and "healthful" are different terms. At the Northwestern University Medical School, heart expert Jeremiah Stamler comments:

> An appropriate standard for normal, based on the vast amount of new information available, is in the range of less than 200 mg per 100 ml. Values of 250 mg per 100 ml or greater are appropriately designated definitely and grossly abnormal, those in the range 200 to 249 are borderline. The old standards need to be discarded and new ones substituted.

Other heart researchers agree—sounding almost like a broken record when asked for their definition of a good cholesterol level.

"Under 200," says Dr. Robert Wissler, the University of Chicago authority on animal atherosclerosis.

"Those of us in nutritional medicine are happier if we can keep our own cholesterol and our patients' in the range of 200 or lower," says Dr. Frederick Stare, retired chairman of Harvard's Nutrition Department.

Some medical sources use not 200, but 220 as the upper limit of "desirable" for the cholesterol level of middle-aged adults. Both the American Medical Association and the National Heart, Lung, and Blood Institute have suggested the slightly higher value as a guideline.

People do vary in their sensitivity to saturated fat and cholesterol, and some who eat the typical American diet will have cholesterol levels below 200 or 220 nonetheless. A majority of American adults, however, do not. About half of American adults have a cholesterol level above 220; sixty percent have levels above 200. Some of those with levels below 220 are young adults who are likely to develop levels above 220 because cholesterol levels rise with age—at least in Western cultures such as our own. Men with blood cholesterol levels of 200 at age twenty are likely to average levels above 250 by middle age. On the other hand, men with levels between 180 and 200 during young adulthood (ages eighteen to thirty-five) will probably average levels in the range of 220 to 230 during middle age. These figures show the importance of considering age when judging cholesterol levels.

Though much has been learned about diet and heart disease, more questions remain to be answered. Some researchers believe that saturated fat and cholesterol have negative effects on the arteries regardless of the blood cholesterol level. Research into this theory is only beginning, but some scientists feel that saturated fat may increase the risk of blood clots in addition to raising blood cholesterol levels. A few studies have shown that cholesterol in foods may have adverse effects on the HDL. Still other studies have found that unsaturated fats may have some effect on the arteries, though for heart disease saturated fat seems more hazardous than unsaturated. These factors have led some scientists to conclude that all individuals should moderately reduce fat and cholesterol to prevent heart disease—with those at highest risk making the biggest cutbacks.

On the other hand, however, is unresolved research showing that in men cholesterol levels below 180 are associated with excess mortality from diseases other than heart disease, including a few forms of cancer. Whether these findings—which have been found in some studies but not in others—mean that low blood cholesterol levels may have adverse effects will not be known for quite some time. Researchers believe that the low cholesterol levels may simply reflect other factors that do increase risk of certain diseases; for instance, a heavy drinker might eat little saturated fat and have low blood cholesterol but would have a much higher than average risk of death because of a high alcohol intake. In one study, those with low blood cholesterol levels also had low levels of vitamin A in their blood—a fact that might explain their excess risk of stomach cancer. It is also possible that cholesterol levels fall when people become ill—meaning that the disease is causing the low cholesterol level, rather than the low cholesterol level causing the disease. Though health authorities have little reason to believe that low blood cholesterol levels actually cause disease, the National Heart, Lung, and Blood Institute has suggested caution in recommending cholesterol-lowering diets to middle-aged men who have blood cholesterol levels below 180 until more is known about these findings. About 12 percent of middle-aged men have levels this low. The NHLBI stresses that the hazards of a low cholesterol level are conjectural, while the hazards of a high cholesterol level are certain.

As we all know, blood cholesterol is not the only influence on heart disease and stroke. Research also indicts high blood pressure and smoking as major risk factors, with high blood pressure the most important risk factor for stroke. Lack of exercise, stress, obesity, and other characteristics also fit into the picture, but are not as serious risk factors as high blood cholesterol, cigarette smoking, and high blood pressure.

What's most interesting is that high blood pressure and

smoking are associated with high rates of heart disease only in countries where blood cholesterol levels are also high. The Japanese eat much less saturated fat than we do, and their cholesterol levels are much lower. But the Japanese have not been as cautious about their use of cigarettes, or of salt—a factor in high blood pressure. Three-fourths of Japanese men smoke, while fewer than half of American men smoke. High blood pressure affects 20 to 30 percent of the Japanese, while in the United States a smaller percentage—about 15 to 20 percent—have high blood pressure. Yet, despite their higher rates of high blood pressure and smoking, Japanese men have only one-sixth the heart attack rate of white American men. Apparently the low cholesterol levels of the Japanese are their savior.

Japan is not an isolated case. Scientists working on the International Atherosclerosis Project found high blood pressure common in Jamaica, but heart attacks rare. The Jamaican diet also had much less saturated fat and cholesterol than our own. Other studies point in the same direction, showing smoking and high blood pressure associated with high rates of heart disease only where high cholesterol levels are common.

It's important to understand what these findings do and do not show. They do show high blood pressure and smoking linked to massive rates of heart disease only in populations that also eat diets high in saturated fat and cholesterol. They do not show that smoking and high blood pressure have *no effect* on a person's atherosclerosis or his risk of heart disease. Smoking and high blood pressure do aggravate atherosclerosis at all levels of cholesterol, but the added effect at low cholesterol levels does not result in atherosclerosis severe enough to cause widespread occurrence of heart attacks. Regardless, high blood pressure contributes to strokes and smoking to lung cancer. *The real value of this knowledge is in its irony; while a diet rich in saturated fat and cholesterol is labeled the most controversial risk factor for heart disease, evidence shows that epidemics of heart attack don't happen without it.*

"It is reasonable and sound," says heart expert Jeremiah Stamler, "to designate 'rich' diet as a primary, essential, necessary cause of the current epidemic of premature atherosclerotic disease raging in the Western and industrialized countries. Cigarette smoking and hypertension [high blood pressure] are important secondary or complementary causes."

At Federal Trade Commission hearings, Dr. Robert Wissler of the University of Chicago told listeners much the same. "I believe that even under conditions where there is widespread presence of other risk factors that you hear about, such as cigarette smoking or hypertension or emotional stress, that these really have very little influence on the [heart] disease except as added factors. In other words, that the primary problem . . . is what is happening in terms of cholesterol," he explained.

At the same hearing, Dr. Mark Hegsted, now director of the federal government's Human Nutrition Center, gave his perspective:

You can't tell anybody that drives 65 miles an hour that they are going to have an accident and kill themselves, but we know the risk of having an accident increases with speed, and therefore, we set some kind of reasonable speed limit. And the situation with regard to diet is exactly the same. You have got a high risk population, and we should begin to modify the diet in terms of what is reasonable.

But some insist that we still don't know enough to act.

4

Arguing Till Doomsday

March 14, 1979, was the centennial of Albert Einstein's birth, and newspapers were alive with tributes to the great physicist and his contributions to science. Sandwiched between explanations of his theories were some human-interest anecdotes; according to one, Einstein had so much trouble remembering which house was his that he painted his front door red. The physicist, it seemed, was an absent-minded professor with brilliant insights into the physical world.

But Einstein's biographers say he was anything but the absent-minded professor; rather, he was an observant man whose insights extended not simply to the physical world but also to human behavior. "Einstein was hardly out of touch with the realities, often grim, of the academic and political world," wrote Richard Smith in *The Washington Post*, relating this encounter between Einstein and another Princeton professor:

Psychologist Hadley Cantril, who lived a few doors away [from Einstein] on Mercer Street, once demonstrated his now-famous trapezoidal room for Einstein. The physicist grasped at once the psychological and philosophical import of the perceptual illusions caused by the seemingly square interior. Dr. Cantril remarked that he was frustrated by the refusal of fellow psychologists to take his findings seriously. Einstein comforted Cantril by noting, "I have learned, don't waste time trying to convince your colleagues."

Einstein was not the only physicist of his time to wonder if words directed at skeptical colleagues weren't words well-wasted. His German colleague, physicist Max Planck, was also struck by the resistance of scientists to new ideas. In his 1936 work, *The Philosophy of Physics,* Planck wrote:

An important scientific innovation rarely makes its way by gradually winning over and converting its opponents: it rarely happens that Saul becomes Paul. What does happen is that its opponents gradually die out and that the growing generation is familiarized with the idea from the beginning.

Planck would find nothing unusual in the heated battle over the causes of heart disease. He would see research linking heart disease to the saturated fat and cholesterol of nutrient-rich foods as a scientific innovation and would regard those who deny its importance as "Sauls" who will never be converted to newer opinions about egg yolk or meat and dairy fat. The Sauls are not only scientists, but threatened farm interests, and no amount of evidence can convince them. "You will be arguing until doomsday on what causes heart attacks," Pennsylvania Senator Richard Schweiker told egg producers.

The litany of ifs, ands, and buts challenging the evidence against saturated fat and cholesterol may never end given the economic problems that the research poses. "Because commercial stakes are enormous, different segments of the food industry select reports and arguments to support their particular interests and bombard us all with propaganda ranging from the most subtle to the crudest claims that governmental regulation may allow," wrote University of Minnesota professor Dr. Ancel

Keys. "It is no wonder that the medical profession is almost as confused as the general public."

Almost twenty years have passed since Keys wrote these words, but arguments against lowering the saturated fat and cholesterol content of our diets are still with us. Just as Keys wrote, powerful farm interests still make certain that every argument is heard. Sometimes, the argument is simply that the facts aren't all in, which is always true in science. But those who use this argument will often recommend other health measures with less evidence than we have against saturated fat and cholesterol. Still other arguments have validity, but not enough to deny the importance of fat and cholesterol. And in some cases, the facts simply don't support the common arguments that we hear:

Argument 1:

Diets lower in saturated fat and cholesterol prevent heart disease, but cause malnutrition instead.

At a Senate hearing in 1977, Dr. Robert Olson, professor at St. Louis University School of Medicine, predicted that diets lower in saturated fat and cholesterol would cause "increased deficiencies of protein, iron, vitamin A, calcium, and riboflavin in vulnerable groups who are not at risk from coronary disease." To illustrate his point, he added, "A low rate of coronary artery disease is associated with those countries that live on cereals. Thailand is an example, where rice is a staple of the diet. Those countries living on cereal grains have a lower rate of coronary heart disease but they also have an enormous rate of malnutrition."

"Going through the line in this cafeteria this noon, how are you going to stop that slim gal up there who took a coke and the

72

little package of cookies for lunch? Now what kind of lunch is that?" University of Illinois professor Dr. Fred Kummerow asked the judge at a Federal Trade Commission hearing where the egg industry had been charged with false advertising. The point was obvious: Eggs are better than junk food.

Of course one can argue that whole milk is better than Coke, or that anyone who eats only rice will develop malnutrition. But whole milk is not the only alternative to Coke, nor is a rice diet the only alternative to hot dogs, butter, and eggs for breakfast every day.

Next to the whole milk in the supermarket are skim and low-fat milks. The only thing whole milk has that the others don't is extra fat and calories. Skim milk provides as much protein, calcium, B vitamins, and other nutrients as whole milk—with 8 fewer grams of fat and 70 to 80 fewer calories per glass.

Like whole milk, fatty meat has nothing that lean meat lacks—except fat and calories. In fact, trimmed meat provides more nutrients than untrimmed cuts. The nutrients in meat concentrate in the muscle of the meat, not in the fat. This means that lean meat has more iron than fatty meat, and iron, of course, is meat's claim to fame.

Meat is an excellent source of iron. Its advantage over other iron-containing foods, however, has been exaggerated by the method used to measure iron. When iron is measured per 100 grams of meat (about 3½ ounces), meat looks like a far better source of iron than other foods. But meat stands out by this standard partly because 100 grams of many meats has more calories than 100 grams of fish or chicken. One hundred grams of untrimmed T-bone steak has 473 calories, while 100 grams of chicken has only 248. Comparing the iron content of the chicken to that of the meat isn't an even trade; you'd have to consider the iron content of the food eaten in addition to the chicken to give as many calories as the steak. For this reason, considering both iron content of meat per 100 calories and per 100 grams is reasonable. On the calorie basis, chicken and fish compare favorably with fatty meats—in fact, they do a little better. Lean meat, however, remains the best source of iron, though a few surprises (such as scallops) crop up.

Club Steak, Cooked, Choice Grade

	Lean with outside fat, 4 ounces	Lean only, 4 ounces
What you don't want		
Calories	515	277
Fat, grams (g)	46	15
What you do want		
Protein, g	23	34
Iron, milligrams (mg)	3	4
Thiamin, mg (vitamin B₁)	.07	.09
Riboflavin, mg (vitamin B₂)	.19	.26
Niacin, mg (vitamin B₃)	4.9	6.6

Source: *Nutritive Value of American Foods,* Agriculture Handbook 456, U.S. Department of Agriculture, 1975.

Iron in Poultry, Fish, and Fatty Meats

	Mg Iron per 100 Calories	Mg Iron per 100 Grams (3½ ounces)
T-bone steak, untrimmed	.5	2.6 (473 calories)
Spare ribs	.6	2.6 (440 calories)
Hot dogs	.5	1.5 (304 calories)
Chicken roasted, with skin	.7	1.8 (248 calories)
Tuna in oil, drained	1.0	1.9 (197 calories)
Flounder, baked with margarine	.7	1.4 (202 calories)
Scallops, steamed	2.7	3 (112 calories)

Iron in Well-Trimmed or Lean Meats

T-bone steak, trimmed of all fat	1.6	3.7 (223 calories)
Flank steak	1.9	3.8 (196 calories)
Pork loin, trimmed of all fat	1.5	3.8 (254 calories)
Leg of lamb, trimmed of all fat	1.2	2.2 (186 calories)

Recently nutritionists have become concerned with the type of iron in foods—not just the total amount. Iron that is bound to the hemoglobin or myoglobin (the form of hemoglobin found in muscle) is the best absorbed form. Nutritionists call this "heme" iron. Beef, chicken, and lamb contain the highest proportion of heme iron—about half the iron in these foods occurs in the heme form. Fish and pork are not far behind, with 40 percent of their iron in the heme form. Other foods contain nonheme iron, but this iron is still useful in the body. The heme iron even seems to help the body better use the nonheme form.

Fish and chicken can not only supply the iron found in fatty meat, but also other meat nutrients. Fish and poultry are good sources of B vitamins and protein, and, in some cases, provide more of these nutrients than fatty meat. Pork is the undisputed champion for thiamin, but natural experiments tell us that thiamin needs can be met by other foods. Religious groups that shun pork aren't known for high rates of beri-beri, the thiamin deficiency disease. They get thiamin from another underrated food: bread.

The emphasis on animal protein that has dominated nutrition for the past half-century has left most of us believing that vegetable foods are only good for vitamins A and C. Food composition tables make clear that this isn't so. The green pea, for instance, has as much protein, vitamin A, and riboflavin as the egg; both contain the same tiny amount of calcium. But the pea contains much more iron, niacin, thiamin, and potassium than the egg—with no cholesterol. The egg may have higher-quality protein, but this is an academic consideration that is rarely of practical importance in diets of adults who consume sufficient calories.

The Incredible, Edible Pea

	1 large egg, hard-boiled	¾ cup green peas, cooked
Calories	82	86
Fat, grams (g)	6	less than 1
Cholesterol, milligrams (mg)	252	0
Protein, g	6	6
Iron, mg	1.2	2.2
Vitamin A, international units (i.u.)	590	645
Thiamin, mg	.04	.34
Riboflavin, mg	.14	.14
Niacin, mg	trace	2.8
Phosphorous, mg	103	118
Calcium, mg	27	28
Vitamin C, mg	0	24
Potassium, mg	65	236

Source: *Nutritive Value of American Foods,* Agriculture Handbook 456, U.S. Department of Agriculture, 1975.

But all this is almost beside the point—a cholesterol-lowering diet doesn't eliminate egg yolk, or dairy fat or meat fat. It simply involves eating less of them. Clearly, this can be done without causing rampant malnutrition.

Argument 2:

Control of obesity—not restriction of saturated fat and cholesterol—is the key to preventing heart disease.

Heart researchers have long wondered where this idea came from. It's not that obesity isn't a risk factor for heart disease. Rather, it's that research does not show obesity to be one of the most important risk factors.

"Obesity is of special interest," writes the National Heart, Lung, and Blood Institute. "Its predictive power in most prospective studies [the best kind] falls considerably short of the major risk factors." The NHLBI ranks obesity as a "suspected" risk factor for heart disease.

Obesity can raise blood cholesterol levels, and is also associated with lower levels of the beneficial HDL-cholesterol. Recommending weight loss as the only measure for controlling high cholesterol won't eliminate the problem, however, because there are people with high cholesterol who have no weight to lose. In addition, there is the problem of feasibility. Heart researchers endorse weight control, but have been disappointed at the outcome of this advice. Opponents of recommendations to eat less saturated fat and cholesterol argue that we should "just lose weight," implying that weight loss is a simple task. Firm statistics are few, but scientists estimate that only 10 percent—20 percent tops—of overweight individuals succeed at losing weight.

Few studies have measured people's willingness to eat less saturated fat and cholesterol, but the results of the experiments so far are a bit more encouraging. In the mid-sixties, the National Diet-Heart Study tested the potential for lowering blood cholesterol by providing specially prepared foods lower in saturated fat and cholesterol to men living otherwise normal lives. Men eating the special foods successfully lowered their cholesterol levels. Nutritionists involved in the experiment estimated that 75 percent of the participants adhered at least fairly well to their new diets. About 20 percent were rated excellent adherers. Most important, a diet with only 30 percent of calories from fat was as well liked as a diet with 40 percent of calories from fat. The *Dietary Goals for the United States* recommends a diet with 30 percent of calories from fat.

National Heart, Lung, and Blood Institute
Report on Risk Factors*

Established Risk Factors

1. High concentration of blood cholesterol—particularly low-density lipoprotein (LDL)
2. High blood pressure
3. Cigarette smoking

Probable Risk Factors

1. Diabetes
2. Stress and coronary-prone behavior
3. Postmenopausal state
4. Family history and genetic factors
5. Contraceptive pills

Suspected Risk Factors

1. Overweight
2. Physical inactivity

Though research has not established obesity as the most serious risk factor for heart disease—nor weight control as the most effective means of controlling blood cholesterol—it's easy to understand why recommending weight loss comes easier than recommending diets lower in saturated fat and cholesterol. "Obesity results from too much food in general rather than too much of one particular food such as meat, milk, or eggs," wrote a group of Iowa farm interests in a paper opposing the *Dietary Goals for the United States*. It's much easier to pass the buck to "too many calories" rather than advocate less of specific foods.

But these efforts to substitute vague recommendations such as "eat fewer calories" for more specific recommendations such as

*From *Arteriosclerosis*, the report of the 1977 working group to review the 1971 report by the National Heart and Lung Institute Task Force on Arteriosclerosis.

"eat fewer high-fat meats and dairy products" paint the two approaches as separate issues. The two couldn't be more closely related. The same diet that raises blood cholesterol also encourages weight gain because foods rich in saturated fat are also high in calories; fat, with more than twice the calories per gram of protein or carbohydrate, is *fattening*. Theoretically, one can gain weight eating too many cucumbers, but realistically, low-fat diets are much less likely to cause weight problems. (This rule does not apply to cholesterol, however; some high-cholesterol foods, such as eggs and shrimp, are low in calories.)

There is no easier way to reduce calories in your diet than to eat less fat. The most successful weight loss program—Weight Watchers—limits calories partly by limiting fat. The Weight Watchers diet allows 30 percent of its calories from fat—the same proportion that the *Dietary Goals* recommends for controlling blood cholesterol levels.

Argument 3:

Lack of exercise is a more important cause of heart disease than diet.

The National Heart, Lung, and Blood Institute's evaluation of inactivity as a risk factor for heart disease was just as surprising as its comments on obesity. "Lack of exercise is generally regarded as a minor factor in the development of atherosclerosis," read the 1977 NHLBI report, *Arteriosclerosis*. The NHLBI placed inactivity in the "suspected" category of risk factors, while eight other factors were given greater emphasis as "established" or "probable" risk factors. "Exercise continues to be promoted as a method to prevent premature heart disease. Its effectiveness is uncertain," says the NHLBI.

Research has found some benefits of exercise. A few studies have shown that vigorous exercise reduces blood cholesterol by

10 percent or more. More commonly, though, the effect of exercise on blood cholesterol levels has been smaller—in the range of a 1 to 3 percent reduction. Recent reports have also found that joggers have higher levels of HDL-cholesterol, a finding that is sure to prompt direct testing of exercise on HDL. Most scientists also believe that exercise helps regulate body weight, which in turn can benefit blood pressure and blood cholesterol.

These benefits notwithstanding, however, lack of exercise still is not as significant as the three major risk factors, and exercise alone is not considered the answer to heart disease. "Physical exercise alone is not enough to counterbalance the incidence of other powerful atherogenic [artery-clogging] traits," concludes Dr. William Kannel, director of the Framingham Heart Study. Among the 4,000 residents of Framingham, Massachusetts, studied by Kannel, a sedentary life-style was associated with higher heart disease rates in men, but not in women. But as is typical, other risk factors were more important than the activity level. "Just throw away your cigarette pack and you've done more than all that jogging," says Kannel.

Results of other exercise studies have been mixed. Some studies do show marked differences in heart disease rates between active and inactive people; a number of studies do not. Interpretation of the studies has been difficult, because exercise habits are rarely the only difference between those who sit and those who don't. "You don't see many fat, smoking joggers," quips William Kannel. Blood cholesterol, blood pressure, and smoking habits often vary among the active and inactive groups. How much of these differences can be attributed to exercise itself is difficult to say.

Those who argue that exercise alone will prevent heart disease often cite the Masai tribe of East Africa. The Masai men live on a diet of meat, milk, and blood, yet their cholesterol levels average less than 150. Scientists do not know why, though a few ideas have been proposed. Most interesting are preliminary findings that fermented milk—which comprises much of the Masai diet—helps to lower blood cholesterol. If this proves true, yogurt should continue to gain popularity. Scientists have also proposed that frequent periods of starvation might help regulate Masai cholesterol.

Some people insist, however, that the Masai experience shows that diets high in saturated fat don't raise blood cholesterol levels. This idea—that an occasional baffling exception invalidates abundant evidence showing a strong relationship between saturated fat and blood cholesterol—will probably not go down in history as brilliant scientific thinking. Those who offer this argument also say that the Masai prove that active life-styles protect against high cholesterol and heart disease. However, another African tribe, the Rendille, lives an active life-style and eats a diet like the Masai. Scientists found blood cholesterol levels in this tribe averaged 233—more than the U.S. average.

The puzzling example of the Masai is matched by another, less-publicized example on the opposite extreme. The farmers and lumberjacks of North Karelia, Finland, live unusually active lives, yet suffer one of the highest heart disease rates in the world. Their diet contains even more saturated fat than our own, and it shows in their average blood cholesterol levels of 270. Obesity is also uncommon among the Karelians, so neither inactivity nor excess weight can explain their plight. For every argument that the Masai prove that exercise is a cure-all, one could argue that the Karelians prove it doesn't help at all. The truth, no doubt, lies somewhere in between.

Argument 4:

Blood cholesterol levels can only be lowered 10 to 15 percent—a trivial amount.

It's true that a 10 to 15 percent lowering of cholesterol levels is what can be expected from the diet recommended by the Senate

Nutrition Subcommittee in its *Dietary Goals for the United States.* That diet looks like this:

Saturated fat	10% of calories
Polyunsaturated fat	10% of calories
Cholesterol	300 mg/day
Total fat	30% of calories

Recommendations from the American Heart Association and other heart disease committees are similar.

Greater reductions of blood cholesterol can be achieved with a stricter diet. The traditional Japanese fish and rice diet, for instance, contains far less saturated fat than the diet proposed in the *Dietary Goals.* The fish and rice diet looks like this:

Saturated fat	3% of calories
Polyunsaturated fat	3% of calories
Cholesterol	300 mg/day
Total fat	10% of calories

On this diet, cholesterol levels would probably drop an average 30 percent. But most nutritionists believe Americans would sooner choose the *Dietary Goals* diet, and if they're right, so are the people who say that a drop in blood cholesterol of 10 to 15 percent is all that we can expect.

The latter group of people is wrong, though, to assume that a 10 to 15 percent reduction in blood cholesterol would have trivial effects on heart disease rates. In 1972, the Inter-Society Commission on Heart Disease Resources issued a comprehensive strategy for preventing heart disease. The Commission had representatives from twenty-nine medical societies, and one task force used results from the on-going Framingham Heart Study to estimate the benefits of lowering cholesterol levels. Their calculations show that the benefits expected far exceed the amount of the reduction. The commission estimated, for instance, that if every American's blood cholesterol level had been 10 percent lower than it was, 24 percent less heart disease would have been expected. If cholesterol levels had been 15 percent lower across the board, the experts predicted that the heart disease caseload would have been 35 percent lighter. The projections, of course, assume long-term lowering of cholesterol levels. They don't promise overnight results.

According to Dr. Robert Levy, director of the National Heart, Lung, and Blood Institute, a 4 to 8 percent fall in average blood cholesterol levels during the last ten years may account for one-third to one-half of the 20 percent fall in heart disease deaths that occurred between 1968 and 1978. We will never know this for sure, but the lessons of that decade may be confirming what the Inter-Society Commission predicted: that small changes in blood cholesterol levels can mean big changes in our heart disease rates.

Argument 5:

If any food causes heart disease, it's refined sugar.

Scientific support for the case against sugar originated with population comparisons published by British researcher Dr. John Yudkin. Yudkin's work showed that populations having high rates of heart disease used large amounts of sugar. It was obvious, though, that the same populations ate diets high in saturated fat, making it impossible to blame sugar with certainty. Heart experts also pointed to a number of countries—for instance, Cuba, Honduras, Costa Rica, and others—where diets were high in sugar but heart disease rates low.

When sugar, a "simple" carbohydrate, is substituted for starch, a "complex" carbohydrate, little change occurs in the blood cholesterol of an average group of people. Some studies have shown a slight increase in blood cholesterol when sugar is substituted for starchy foods, but this may reflect a slight cholesterol-lowering effect of the fiber in the starches. Compared to the effect of saturated fat and cholesterol, the effect of sugar has been at most small.

Though sugar does not seem to affect blood cholesterol in most people, a subgroup of people may be unusually sensitive to it. In one recent study with people who showed atypical insulin reactions to sugar, sugar raised cholesterol levels. Sugar also raises blood triglyceride levels in a minority of people. The National Heart, Lung, and Blood Institute says that the relationship between blood triglycerides and heart disease remains uncertain; current thinking holds that high blood triglycerides may simply reflect other risk factors directly linked to heart disease, such as low levels of HDL-cholesterol, and high total blood cholesterol levels. Nonetheless, the NHLBI does recommend restriction of sugar for individuals with high triglyceride levels.

Even though research has never established sugar as a cause of heart disease in the general population, eating less of it is a good idea. As we all know, sugar is a major cause of tooth decay. Today, it supplies 20 percent of the calories in the average American diet, lowering our intake of nutritious foods by about that amount.

Argument 6:

Women can eat as much saturated fat and cholesterol as they want until menopause.

Through middle age, women are blessed with remarkably less heart disease than men. White American men aged thirty-five to fifty-four are five times as likely to die from heart disease as white women. Black men also suffer more heart disease deaths during these years than black women, but the differences are not as great as among whites. After age fifty-five, the gap between sexes narrows, and late in life, the women catch up with the men.

The good fortune of women has led to the optimistic assumption that women are immune to atherosclerosis until later life. Some also assume that women have low cholesterol levels until menopause, which usually occurs between the ages of forty-five and fifty.

American women have lower cholesterol levels than American men only during the ages of twenty-five to forty-four. During this time, cholesterol levels of American women average 7 to 15 mg lower than the men's average—a significant, but not enormous, difference. Relative to men around the globe, however, these "lower" levels are not "low." Men in Tanushimaru, Japan, average cholesterol levels of 170 between the ages of forty and fifty-nine; American women average this level when they are twelve years old. In the Italian cities of Crevalcore and Montegiorgio, middle-aged men average levels of 195. American women reach this average level twenty years earlier. At the same level of total blood cholesterol level, however, women generally have more of the beneficial HDL-cholesterol than men.

If women were immune to atherosclerosis until menopause, as some claim, their cholesterol levels would be irrelevant. The hormone estrogen, secreted by women until menopause, may have some beneficial effect on the arteries. The small amount of information available, however, does not show women to be free of serious atherosclerosis until menopause. In the International Atherosclerosis Project, scientists documented noteworthy differences in the amount of plaque among 3,000 deceased women from different areas of the world. As with the men, the amount of plaque varied considerably from country to country. In the United States, white women aged thirty-five to forty-four had three times as much severe plaque as women of the same age living in less-developed nations. In every country but one, women did have less atherosclerosis than the men in their communities. (American black women had as much advanced atherosclerosis as American black men.) But though younger women generally had less atherosclerosis than the men in their own communities, premenopausal women in some areas had more atherosclerosis than men who lived in other parts of the world.

Not surprisingly, the heart disease rates of women parallel these findings. Women do have heart attacks before menopause, but at a rate far lower than the men in that same country. When comparisons are made among countries, however, the story changes. White American women aged thirty-five to fifty-four are 1.5 to 2 times as likely to die of heart disease as Japanese men of the same age. Yet, American women smoke far less and have less high blood pressure than the Japanese men. The higher cholesterol levels of American women stand accused.

Death Rates from Heart Disease
per 100,000 People, 1973*

	Ages 35–44	Ages 45–54
Japanese women	2.8	11.3
Japanese men	9.5	30.7
U.S. women (white)	14.6	65.8
U.S. men (white)	75.4	312.9

The knowledge about women and heart disease shows that atherosclerosis does develop in women before menopause, but because it develops at a slower rate than in men, complications do not set in until later in life. One can argue both sides for what premenopausal women should do. On one hand, one could say that women should not let their cholesterol levels rise during the premenopausal years, for when menopause occurs, they will be left with the high cholesterol level but not the protection against rapid accumulation of plaques. (Some scientists believe that once

*Source: National Heart, Lung, and Blood Institute, unpublished data.

cholesterol levels are high, getting them down may be more difficult than maintaining a lower level all through life—but no one knows for sure.) On the other hand, one can argue that women can eat more saturated fat and cholesterol than men until menopause because the same diet is not as potent a risk factor for them. Obviously, "more is permissible" does not mean any amount is desirable.

The debate becomes almost moot, however, when one looks beyond the issue of heart disease and considers all the effects of our present diet. American women do not have high rates of heart disease before menopause, but they are more likely than men to be plagued by obesity. As far as calories are concerned, a high-fat diet is the worst, for nothing makes the calories add up as quickly as fat does. In addition, American women suffer high rates of breast and colon cancers, and our high-fat diet is the prime suspect. Findings from several types of studies suggest that for breast cancer, life-style and environment during early life— particularly during the teens—influence risk most strongly. When the whole picture is considered, a lower fat diet makes good advice for younger women as well as men. The major difference is that all fats are suspect for cancers and, of course, for obesity, whereas for heart disease, reducing saturated fat is more important.

Argument 7:

There is no proof that lowering blood cholesterol levels will prevent heart disease.

For twenty years, heart researchers have invested time and money in search of the final piece of evidence: evidence that lowering blood cholesterol levels will do what we presume they will—lessen our risk of heart disease. The devil's advocate loves to insist that we cannot assume that lower cholesterol levels won't mean less heart disease simply because it is a fact that where cholesterol levels are low, heart disease is rare, or because animal evidence and what we know about diet and cholesterol levels point to the very same conclusion.

Heart researchers use the term "intervention study" to describe that last piece of evidence that would prove the point. An intervention study is one where cholesterol levels are lowered among a group of people, and their heart attack rates are compared to another group not given the same cholesterol-lowering treatment.

More than a dozen intervention studies, from small to medium in size, have been conducted during the past twenty years. Some of the opponents of dietary change insist that the results have been negative. But the intervention studies cannot be lumped together. About half, for instance, involved heart attack survivors, and in one of these studies researchers found that once a heart attack has occurred the most important factor influencing future heart health was the severity of the prior heart attack(s). High blood cholesterol remained a risk factor for the heart attack survivors, but only a modest one. By contrast, high blood cholesterol is a powerful risk factor before a heart attack occurs.

Some of the intervention studies lowered cholesterol not with diet but with drugs. Obviously, the two approaches are not exactly the same. Though both drugs and diets lower in saturated fat and cholesterol lower blood cholesterol levels, the mode of action in the body is not the same. Drugs also have side effects that a diet lower in fat is not known to have. (A diet high in polyunsaturated fat, however, may produce toxic effects similar to certain cholesterol-lowering drugs.)

Experiments with heart attack survivors and/or drugs account for many of the intervention studies done so far. Only a few have tested the effect of cholesterol-lowering diets on subjects who have never suffered a heart attack. Scientists constantly argue about the soundness of each one, but two are generally acknowledged as the best of the lot: the Los Angeles Veterans study and the Finnish Hospital study. The Los Angeles study reported forty-eight deaths attributed to atherosclerosis among the men who followed a cholesterol-lowering diet and seventy due to atherosclerosis in men who ate the typical American diet. The difference was statistically significant and most noticeable in the younger half of the group, men aged fifty-four to sixty-five. In the old half, men aged sixty-six to eighty-eight, the effect on diseases attributed to atherosclerosis was small, underscoring the need to act earlier in life. The Finnish Mental Hospital study reported similar results for men. Men on a cholesterol-lowering diet had half as much heart disease as men who ate the typical Finnish diet rich in dairy fats. Women also had less heart disease on the cholesterol-lowering diet, but the difference was not statistically significant. The results do not sit with the assertion that "there is no evidence that lowering cholesterol will prevent heart attacks."

The more baffling question is how to interpret the intervention studies, because a statistically significant effect on all causes of death was not found. In the Los Angeles study, total deaths were similar in both groups. In Finland, fewer deaths occurred in the group of men on the cholesterol-lowering diet, but the effect was not statistically significant—perhaps because too few subjects were involved. (When few subjects are involved, more dramatic differences are needed to show statistical significance.) In women, no differences in total mortality were found, but again, the number of deaths was small. The results have not surprised some researchers, who believe that the total fat content of the diet needs to be reduced. In studies done so far, researchers didn't lower all fats; they substituted polyunsaturated fat for saturated fat. But today, health professionals recommend eating less of all fats. The *Dietary Goals for the United States,* for instance, recommends not just a substitution of unsaturated for saturated fat, but a 25 percent decrease in total fat intake. Researchers are also wary of diets very high in polyunsaturated fat—precisely the kind used in Los Angeles and Finland.

Only a few studies with low-fat diets have been reported, and not one comes close to meeting today's standards for an intervention experiment. All are very small. Scientists simply told the patients what to eat; they did not control their diets as was the case in Los Angeles or Finland. But the results do show that the effects of a diet lower in all fats should be studied.

• Dr. Lester Morrison reported that 19 of 50 patients asked to follow a diet very low in fat lived for twelve years, while none of the 50 not asked to follow such a diet survived this long.

• Dr. Thomas Lyon and his colleagues reported that recurrence of heart attack and death was four times as common in patients who admitted they were not adhering to the very low-fat diet prescribed by the doctors.

• Dr. A. Koranyi reported a study of 125 patients asked to follow a diet very low in fat. The death rate in the low-fat group was 9 percent, compared to 19 percent among patients not asked to restrict their fat intake.

Scientists point out that not just these three studies, but all the studies done so far have been too small—hardly large enough to give conclusive answers about specific diseases or total mortality.

Aside from the issue of lowering total fat is another problem. Even the best intervention studies are destined to suffer from a serious drawback—the problem of "too little and too late." To be practical, intervention studies rely heavily on middle-aged or elderly subjects. But middle-aged men and elderly men are likely to have quite a bit of atherosclerosis already. In 1971, the National Heart, Lung, and Blood Institute's Task Force on Arteriosclerosis lamented, "Even in those dietary trials carried out with older subjects free of clinical disease [e.g., a heart attack or angina pectoris], it is known that in most subjects arterial lesions have progressed to the irreversible stage." Dr. Thomas Dawber of Boston Univeristy comments, "It is not reasonable to expect that changes in dietary intake after forty or fifty years on a diet high in fat and cholesterol would produce dramatic results."

But a study with young people is out of the question. A committee convened by the NHLBI during the 1960s concluded that such a study would require at least 50,000 people followed for 10 to 30 years. The cost for such a study would be prohibitive—probably in the billions of dollars. Instead, the NHLBI opted for experiments using both drugs and diet or subjects with more than one risk factor for heart disease. It is hoped that these studies will yield some information about diet, but the NHLBI acknowledges that they may not.

Until more research is available, it's hard to swallow the argument that we shouldn't make judgments based on what we already know. For other risk factors, notably obesity and exercise, one rarely hears intervention studies demanded before recommendations are made. In 1980, the Food and Nutrition Board of the National Academy of Sciences scoffed at recommendations to eat less fat and cholesterol but endorsed weight control, salt restriction, and physical activity. Intervention studies to show that these measures improve life expectancy not only don't exist, but the Food and Nutrition Board didn't even suggest they were necessary. In the case of these risk factors, population studies showing higher risk of disease among obese and inactive people—along with evidence that weight loss can affect risk factors such as blood cholesterol and glucose tolerance (a factor in diabetes)—were enough. The same kind of evidence (plus more) exists for fat and cholesterol. We know that populations eating diets high in saturated fat and cholesterol have high rates of heart disease. We know high blood cholesterol is a risk factor, and we know that saturated fat and cholesterol affect that risk factor.

Heart researchers who advocate diets lower in saturated fat and cholesterol are simply making a judgment based on the large amount of evidence available, and as Dr. Mark Hegsted points out, the Food and Nutrition Board does the same thing for its Recommended Dietary Allowances for the various nutrients. For the most part, the RDAs are based on short-term experiments, not long-term studies. "No proof is available that the RDAs are optimal," says Hegsted, pointing out that for some nutrients, recommended allowances have been formulated with far less evidence than available for saturated fat and cholesterol. "I find it truly amazing," he wrote, "that the Food and Nutrition Board apparently knows enough about human needs to establish recommended allowances for zinc, selenium, and practically all essential nutrients, yet finds insufficient evidence to make recommendations about fat, sugar, cholesterol, and salt. The fact, of course, is that a decision to establish an allowance is not based on the extent of our knowledge but rather on the belief that we need an RDA."

And perhaps the ingrained idea that the RDA for each nutrient is all we need for good health explains why a few unrelenting critics set far higher standards for diets lower in saturated fat and cholesterol than for other commonly accepted health measures.

Argument 8:

We are a healthy people. Proposals for dietary change are the work of hypochondriacs.

Those who dismiss recommendations for a lower fat diet are quick to quote an opening statement in *Healthy People,* the Surgeon General's report that suggested that Americans eat less saturated fat and cholesterol. "The health of the American people has never been better," said the report. So why should we tinker with our diet?

Though life expectancy from birth has increased dramatically in the United States since the turn of the century, this figure can be misleading. Prevention of diseases that kill infants and children greatly increases a nation's total life expectancy, because by preventing these diseases, many decades are added to individuals' lives. Elimination of most childhood diseases and improvement in the infant mortality rate have accounted for most of the increase in life expectancy since the turn of the century. In 1900, a man who survived through childhood and adolescence to age forty, for instance, could have expected to live another 31.2 years.

In 1970, a forty-year-old man could have expected to live another 31.7 years, an improvement of only six months. In other words, we have greatly improved the health status of infants and children, but not of adults. "Whatever social affluence and medicine achieved something else has taken away; that something else is principally the atherosclerotic, coronary, and cardiovascular disease epidemic," comments Dr. Henry Blackburn, heart researcher at the University of Minnesota. Of the 650,000 people who die each year from coronary heart disease, 150,000 are under the age of sixty-five. These figures, of course, consider only death, and not the quality of life. Pain and disability from survived heart attacks, angina pectoris, or other complications of atherosclerosis are difficult to measure.

The argument that "our health is good, so why complain," also assumes that we can judge the effects of our present diet by our current rates of various diseases. But degenerative diseases develop slowly over many years. People who are now old enough to succumb to degenerative diseases have not always eaten as we do now. The fat content of the national food supply, for instance, increased substantially in the early 1940s, again in the late 1960s, and again in the early 1970s. We cannot assume that the long-term effects of these increases, particularly the last two, will be obvious today.

The Surgeon General did say that our health is good. He did not say that it couldn't be better.

Argument 9:
Changing our diet could be risky.

No one can deny the theory behind this argument—that change, by its very definition, brings the possibility of risk.

But as for risks associated with eating a lower-fat diet, none are known. "There is no known evidence that low-cholesterol diets are harmful, or that dietary cholesterol is an essential nutrient in any human condition," concluded a task force of the American Society for Clinical Nutrition, a professional organization of nutrition scientists. The task force on fat reached similar conclusions. "There is no evidence that a low-fat diet is harmful, per se," said the group. In Japan, diets low in saturated fat and cholesterol are associated with life expectancies better than our own, another consolation to those who fear hazards.

Emphasizing the chance of risk ignores two fundamental questions: Is our current diet free of risk? Was it scientifically designed after careful long-term studies? "I think we ought to recognize that the menu we happen to eat today was never planned," Dr. Mark Hegsted told the Federal Trade Commission. "It just grew, like Topsy, as the result of our affluence and the efficiency of the American farmer, and the fact that we consume it today is obviously no indication that it is desirable." With no proof that our current diet is the world's best, and good reason to believe that it isn't, it's a matter of deciding whether to try something else.

The critics of lower-fat diets warn that we could end up with something worse instead, forgetting another important truth about change. Change brings not only harms, but benefits. And in the case of eating less fat, the great majority of heart experts are convinced that the scales are tipped heavily toward the likelihood of benefits.

5

The Illusion of Controversy

The evidence that diet contributes to heart disease has ruffled many feathers and, in return, has been called many names. *People* magazine described the evidence as "puzzling." An egg industry lobbyist called it "unsettled." Dr. George Mann of Vanderbilt University called the low-cholesterol diet "fund-raising propaganda" for the American Heart Association. Most commonly, though, the adjective is "controversial," and if the average person knows nothing else about diet and heart disease, he or she knows the idea is "controversial."

"Every scientific advancement that has been made is controversial," Senator Richard Schweiker has said. There are more than a few nutritionists who don't think that cholesterol-lowering diets qualify for the term "advancement," and in nutrition circles a controversy remains over recommendations to limit meat and milk fats and egg yolk in the diet. But among researchers who have never cherished meat, milk, and eggs in quite the way that nutritionists have, the dissenters are few.

"Like other groups of mortals, scientists are an imperfect and varied lot," Dr. John Olney, professor at Washington University, told a Senate committee in 1969. Recognizing their individual shortcomings, scientists have long studied problems in groups rather than rely on the pronouncement of individuals alone. Committees, no doubt, also have their shortcomings, but are nonetheless trusted as the best source of judgment on important issues.

It was in 1958, fifty years after a Russian scientist made history by producing atherosclerosis in rabbits fed a high-fat, high-cholesterol diet, that a private group, the National Health Education Committee, issued the first scientific statement favoring dietary changes to prevent heart disease. Cautious optimism flavored the statement, for its signers—eight prominent physicians and 106 members of the American Society for the Study of Arteriosclerosis—were sticking their necks out. "The reduction or control of fat consumption under medical supervision, with reasonable substitution of polyunsaturated for saturated fats is recommended as a possible means of preventing heart attacks and strokes," read the statement. It carried a qualification. "This recommendation is based on the best scientific information available at the present time."

Three years later, in 1961, the National Health Education Committee got some company: the American Heart Association. In the first of its many public statements about diet, the Heart Association wrote: "Research studies have given clues to the prevention of atherosclerosis by dietary means. A reduction in blood cholesterol . . . may lessen the development or extension of atherosclerosis and hence the risk of heart attacks or strokes." The Heart Association, too, tempered its recommendation with a warning: "It must be emphasized that there is yet no final proof that heart attacks or strokes will be prevented by such measures."

The researchers went back to their laboratories, continuing investigations into the causes of heart disease. The sixties were an exciting time for researchers, for during this decade evidence confirming the suspected role of saturated fat and cholesterol started pouring in. The guarded tone of earlier pronouncements began to fade. In 1968, the governments of Finland, Sweden, and Norway issued official recommendations for combatting heart disease through diet. Their advice—more fruits, vegetables, potatoes, skim milk, lean meat, fish, and cereal products—was nothing original, but such a message coming from government health officials was a first.

Nineteen sixty-eight was the turning point. The first three official recommendations calling for a new definition of "good nutrition" spanned a decade, but after 1968, a groundswell of agreement emerged. In the following ten years, not three, but sixteen expert committees joined the forces advocating a change in eating habits. Among the new voices were the Task Force on Arteriosclerosis of the National Heart, Lung, and Blood Institute; the White House Conference on Food, Nutrition, and Health; and the World Health Organization.

The twentieth recommendation appeared in 1979, and it was one of the most important, for it bore the seal of Dr. Julius Richmond, the U.S. Surgeon General. In *Healthy People: The Surgeon General's Report on Health Promotion and Disease Prevention*, the nation's top health official endorsed the diet that some of his colleagues had recommended twenty years before. "Americans would probably be healthier, as a whole, if they con- sumed . . . less saturated fat and cholesterol," said the report. A foreword by HEW Secretary Joseph Califano said the report represented "an emerging consensus among the scientists and the health community that the nation's health strategy must be dramatically recast to emphasize the prevention of disease."

An informal survey taken not long before the release of the Surgeon General's report backed the claim of an "emerging consensus" about the role of diet in heart disease. Dr. Kaare Norum of the University of Oslo School of Medicine polled 200 scientists who had attended heart disease conferences, asking their opinions about diet. *A full 92 percent of the respondents favored advising the public to adopt new eating patterns.* The most common recommendation was fewer calories, followed by less saturated fat, less cholesterol, and less total fat. Nine out of ten said they had changed their own eating habits. After the survey was completed, two of this country's most respected nutritionists,

Drs. Jean Mayer and Johanna Dwyer, commented: "It seems clear that this group of eminent international experts agrees with the dietary goals proposed for Americans. And the contention that there are big differences of opinion among the experts is a false one."

There are some differences, however, among the more than twenty expert statements favoring cholesterol-lowering diets. Some statements recommend increases in polyunsaturated fat, while others recommend only restriction of saturated fat and cholesterol. A few make no recommendation on food cholesterol, though the great majority do, just as a few also make no recommendation on limiting the total amount of fat in the diet. But in general, the theme is less fat and cholesterol—especially less saturated fat.

The Growth of a Consensus: Endorsers of Cholesterol-Lowering Diets

1958   National Health Education Committee (U.S.)

1961   American Heart Association

1968   Scandinavian government medical boards (Finland, Sweden, and Norway)

1970   Inter-Society Commission on Heart Disease Resources (U.S.)

1971   Task Force on Arteriosclerosis/National Heart, Lung, and Blood Institute (U.S.)

National Heart Foundation of New Zealand

1972   American Health Foundation

American Medical Association/National Academy of Sciences Food and Nutrition Board

1973   International Society of Cardiology

National Advisory Council on Nutrition of The Netherlands

Report of the 1969 White House Conference on Food, Nutrition, and Health

1974   National Heart Foundation of Australia

United Kingdom Department of Health and Social Security

1975   California Society of Pediatric Cardiology/California Heart Association

Australian Academy of Science

Federal Republic of Germany Report

1976   Royal College of Physicians of London/British Cardiac Society

New Zealand Royal Society

1977   Food and Agriculture Organization/World Health Organization

Quebec Department of Social Affairs

1979   Surgeon General of the United States

1980   U.S. Department of Agriculture/Department of Health
and Human Services

All expert panels except the American Medical Association/National Academy of Sciences report give advice to the general public. Specifics vary from report to report, but the overall theme is less fat, less saturated fat, less cholesterol, and partial replacement of saturated fat with polyunsaturated fat.

All but one of the committees suggest that the general public follow their recommendations. Some object, claiming that cholesterol-lowering diets should be recommended only to those at high risk of heart disease. But because a majority of Americans are at considerable risk of developing heart disease—and also because many Americans do not have their cholesterol levels checked regularly, most committees feel that advice to the general public is warranted. This does not mean that the recommendations are rigid rules that are applicable to every individual, but rather that the guidelines are a general approach advisable for the average person. The Basic Four, after all, was no more than a general approach suitable for many, but hardly all, Americans. And the Recommended Dietary Allowances, the nutrient standards on which the Basic Four is based, are actually higher than necessary for more than 95 percent of the population. The RDA are set high enough to insure nutrient adequacy for all, because determining individual nutrient needs and tailoring every diet accordingly is impossible. Recommendations to the general public regarding fat and cholesterol are based on the same belief: that for practical purposes, a general approach is needed.

The American Medical Association, as well as individual scientists, has taken exception to the general approach to saturated fat and cholesterol. The AMA does endorse the suggestion that Americans should avoid too much of all fats, but declines to endorse advice on saturated fat and cholesterol as a general measure. The AMA does not, however, deny the role of saturated fat and cholesterol in heart disease. In 1972, the group adopted its official position on diet and heart disease, which stated, "The average level of plasma lipids (cholesterol) in most American men and women is undesirably elevated. . . . The evidence now available is sufficient to discourage further temporizing with this major national health problem." For those at high risk—which the statement seems to define as individuals with cholesterol levels above 220—the AMA recommended diets lower in saturated fat and cholesterol. By this definition, half of American adults should be following the AMA's advice. The AMA's statement on diet was cosigned by another group of scientists: the Food and Nutrition Board of the National Academy of Sciences. As of 1979 there had not been a single scientific committee to issue a contrary opinion doubting the role of diet in heart disease.

Then suddenly in 1980, the Food and Nutrition Board, which had earlier said that average blood cholesterol levels were "undesirably elevated" and that evidence was sufficient to act, issued a report called *Toward Healthful Diets,* which scoffed at the more than twenty scientific statements on diet and heart disease. The board charged that these statements "often lack a sound scientific foundation," and went on to assure that "healthy" Americans need not concern themselves with fat and cholesterol. "High-risk" individuals, said the new report, should see their doctors. (The board didn't realize that seemingly "healthy" people are often at high risk of heart disease, since atherosclerosis is a silent process that often shows no ill effects until a heart attack strikes.)

It seemed unexplainable. No new studies directly testing the effect of diet on incidence of heart disease had been published since the 1972 Food and Nutrition Board statement that strongly supported the relationship between diet and heart disease. If there was an explanation for the sudden reversal, it was not that the facts had changed but that membership on the Food and Nutrition Board had changed. In 1980 the board was the personification of nutrition's old school. Most of its members were nutrient specialists; one was an anthropologist. Only one or two were heart researchers, and at that were those that shared a minority viewpoint. Because the board members themselves decide who their members will be, constructing a one-sided committee of scientists who embrace the same viewpoint was simple enough. After *Dietary Goals for the United States* was published in 1977, the one board member who worked on the report was not renominated, while new members added were outspoken critics of the *Dietary Goals*. Two board members—chairman Dr. Alfred Harper and Dr. Robert Olson—were so opposed to the link between diet and heart disease that they served as consultants to the dairy and egg industries. Their belief that foods such as meat, milk, and eggs could not be a major cause of heart disease was so strong that *Toward Healthful Diets* confidently asserted that heart disease is "not primarily nutritional" at the same time that it called the causes of atherosclerosis "unknown" and "poorly understood." It was telling that the board recommended weight control, exercise, and salt restriction without the evidence demanded of fat and cholesterol.

Farm interests, of course, hailed the new report as the work of the most authoritative body in the country. *The New York Times,* on the other hand, described the Food and Nutrition Board as a "group whose objectivity and aptitude are in doubt." *The Washington Post* and many heart scientists criticized the report as inconsistent and lacking in important facts. The Surgeon General and other government health officials stood by their advice to eat less fat and cholesterol.

In general, the board's effort to return nutrition to the days when the only things that mattered were the Recommended Dietary Allowances and weight control (and now salt) was not very successful. It wasn't simply because, the Food and Nutrition Board notwithstanding, medical researchers had reached a consensus that diets high in saturated fat and cholesterol do contribute to heart disease. A growing number of scientists were also concerned that the diet long considered the world's best was, in fact, contributing to high rates of certain cancers.

6

Cancers of Affluence?

"There is a problem in science sometimes that obvious truths sit and wait to be retold," Dr. Robert Levy, director of the National Heart, Lung, and Blood Institute told senators in 1979. Levy and his colleagues in heart research have witnessed it firsthand; the 1908 findings of atherosclerosis in animals fed meat fat, milk fat and egg yolk lay fallow in science journals for years—all but ignored while scientists focused their research on infectious diseases and nutritional deficiencies. And now the cancer researchers are faced with this centuries-old problem. They, too, ignored research linking diet with certain forms of cancer.

For more than a decade, the words *diet* and *cancer* mentioned in the same sentence brought food additives to mind. Any ingredient with a name ten syllables long aroused suspicion, and not without reason. Over the years, the Food and Drug Administration has banned more than twenty-five food additives that proved toxic to man or animals. Fully half of the banned additives have been coal tar dyes, usually known by the euphemism "artificial colors." Though many food additives are safe, scientists doubt

103

that all are, and none are as suspect as the rainbow of artificial colors originally derived from coal tar.

Tar and its derivatives have long been considered toxic substances. But the first clue that food additives such as coal tar dyes were not the only suspicious substances in food dates back half a century—ironically, to one of the coal tar experiments. In 1930, Drs. A. F. Watson and Edward Mellanby treated the skin of two groups of mice with coal tar. Some of the animals were fed high-fat diets, while others were not. The mice fed a diet rich in butter developed twice as many tumors as mice fed a diet low in fat. The tumors, though, were skin tumors, and as sunlight is considered the major factor in human skin cancer, no one is sure that these results apply to man.

But Watson and Mellanby were followed by the classic experiments of Dr. Albert Tannenbaum. In a series of experiments, Tannenbaum found that fat promoted other kinds of cancer in mice—notably breast cancer. After experimenting with protein, calories, and fat, Tannenbaum concluded that fat had the most dramatic effect on breast cancer. In 1942, he wrote:

> The definite increase in the incidence of spontaneous breast tumors brought about by a fat-enriched diet is significant, and this effect is the most striking result obtained in our studies with various types of tumors.

Other researchers experimenting in the 1940s and 1950s confirmed Tannenbaum's findings that fat promoted breast cancer, but for some reason, the information never went too far. The public never heard it, and the scientists more or less ignored it. By the 1950s, cancer research focused on finding a virus that causes cancer and finding a cure for the disease.

Why science allowed its knowledge about fat to collect dust in the library, no one knows, but Dr. Donald Fredrickson, director of the National Institutes of Health (NIH), has dared to guess. At a Senate hearing in 1978, a puzzled George McGovern and his colleague Robert Dole asked Fredrickson why the NIH was spending only 1 percent of its cancer dollars on nutrition when evidence had implicated diet in far more than 1 percent of cancer cases. Fredrickson startled his listeners with this reply:

> The major thing that moves science today is technical opportunity. Immunology has moved like a rocket because there are techniques for measuring antibodies and their relationship to disease and to health. And when we get techniques for measuring nutritional status that are far more microscopic than they are in regard to whether you had a coronary or you have a tumor of the bowel, then we will begin to see movement there, too. And that is the crucial thing that determines the movement in science.

In Fredrickson's view, the opportunities to study the effect of diet on cancer were about as exciting as a dead rat; it simply meant feeding animals different diets and examining them for tumors. The lure of exotic cellular studies with viruses was more tantalizing. And perhaps this is why the dull but promising knowledge about diet and cancer was packed into the crawl spaces of cancer research, and stored there, unopened, for almost two decades.

Were it not for the epidemiologist, the laboratory scientists might never have rescued that box full of experiments showing that fat promotes cancer. Epidemiologists are little impressed with the latest in scientific machinery—or, as Fredrickson put it, "technical opportunity." Rather, they are interested in associations between life-style and disease. Midway into the 1960s, British epidemiologist A. J. Lea found that cancers of the breast and ovaries that occurred after age fifty-five were strongly correlated with the amount of "visible" fat in the diet—that is, obvious fat such as butter, margarine, and vegetable oil. Other epidemiologists picked up from there. Later and more detailed studies, spanning up to forty countries worldwide, confirmed that the total amount of fat in the diet does correlate with some forms of cancer. Studies link six forms of cancer with dietary fat, including cancers of the breast and colon, two of the top cancer killers in the United States. In 1978, 34,000 American women died from breast cancer; and about 42,000 men and women died from colon cancer. In the epidemiological surveys, cancers of the ovary, uterus, prostate gland, and pancreas also correlate with dietary fat.

Comparing fat consumption to cancer rates around the world is the basic form of epidemiology. Another kind of epidemiological research—the study of migrating populations—has also yielded important findings. No culture has offered more opportunity for migrant studies than Japan. Countless Japanese have left their native country to settle in the United States. Both countries have long been industrialized, making it unlikely that problems created by industrialization would explain differences in cancer rates. What's more, Japan's health care system is first-class, giving scientists confidence in the cancer rates reported by Japanese doctors.

Studies of Japanese immigrants tell the same story that was told for heart disease—that environment outstrips heredity as a factor in both diseases. Japanese who leave Japan say good-bye to the high rates of stomach cancer that plague their native land, but after settling in the United States are more likely to develop cancers of the breast, colon, pancreas, uterus, prostate, and ovary than the Japanese natives. Other migrant groups—Polish, Norwegian, Italian, and others—have also shown higher rates of some cancers on immigrating to the United States. But the Japanese findings are the most compelling, for two reasons. First, the number of people studied is large, and second, the diet they left behind is well-known to be very different from our own. Studies of the migrants' dietary habits have found that they compromise on arriving in the United States, retaining some of their native food habits while adopting some of the U.S. menu. The fat content of their diets increases as a result.

A third type of epidemiology—the epidemiology of wealth—has also produced evidence supporting the relationship of fat and cancer. Within the United States, rich and poor alike eat high-fat

Cancers of Affluence?

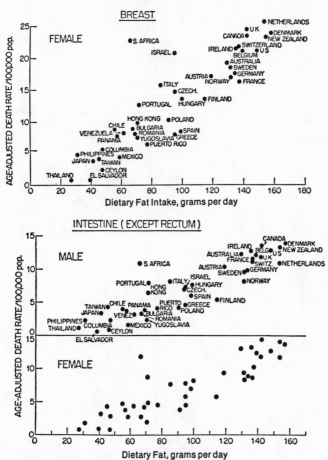

Figure 6: The international correlations between fat intake and cancers of the breast and colon.* In general, rates of these cancers increase with the amount of fat in the diet. South Africa and Israel appear to be exceptions to the trend, but a closer look shows that they are not. The figures for cancer rates in these two countries represent only the white or Jewish populations, while the fat intake is based on the entire country. If the cancer rates included the entire populations of these countries, they would fit into the graphs more closely.

*Graphs courtesy of Drs. K. K. Carroll and H. T. Khor, University of Western Ontario. Published in *Progress in Biochemistry and Pharmacology,* 1975. Reprinted with permission of S. Karger AG, Basel, Switzerland.

107

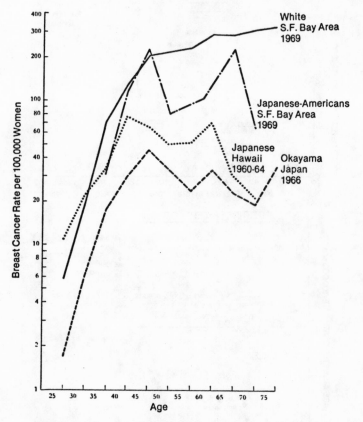

Figure 7: Changes in breast cancer incidence in migrating Japanese women.*
Japanese women who moved to Hawaii had higher rates than women
in the native land, and Japanese-Americans in San Francisco had even
higher rates.

diets, and only the source of that fat (butter versus lard; expensive
meat versus inexpensive) varies. In other parts of the world,
however, the poor are so poor that they cannot even afford the
cheapest meats, and as a result, the poor eat much less fat than the
rich. These nations provide a good testing ground for the
epidemiology of diet and cancer.

*Graph courtesy of Philip Buell, published in *Journal of the National Cancer
Institute,* November 1975.

The upper class of Cali, Colombia, enjoys a high-fat diet uncharacteristic of the lower classes, and with this diet comes a four times greater risk of colon cancer. The upper class in Cali eats more beef, more pork, more eggs, more milk, and more cooking oil than the poorest classes; the only major source of fat that the poor use more of is lard. The extra lard is not enough to bring the poor man's fat intake even close to the fat content of the upper class diet.

Hong Kong has taught us similar lessons about the epidemiology of cancer. In a novel approach to health and wealth,

Breast and Colon Cancers: The Evidence Against Fat

	Breast (Women)	Colon
Incidence, per 100,000 people U.S. whites	74	27 (men) 23 (women)
Incidence, per 100,000 people Japan	14	6 (men) 5 (women)
U.S. vs. Japanese rate	Five times as common in U.S.	Five times as common in U.S.
Japanese immigrant experience	Higher risk on immigrating to U.S., but not as high as U.S. rates for first two generations.	Higher risk on immigrating. For men, almost complete, rapid transition from low Japanese rate to high U.S. rate.

	Breast (Women)	Colon
Other immigrant findings	Polish, German, Norwegian, Irish, English, Swedish and Italian women had higher risk after settling in U.S.	Polish immigrants had higher risk after settling in U.S.
Correlations with fat intake?	Strong worldwide correlation in at least three studies.	Strong worldwide correlation in at least three studies.
Animal experiments	Fat increases breast tumors in mice and rats.	Fat increases risk of chemically induced colon tumors in mice and rats.
Other suspected or known risk factors	Late age at first pregnancy Radiation Family history	Ulcerative colitis Intestinal polyps High meat intake Diet low in fiber

researchers there traced cancer victims back to the street where they lived. They found that people who died of breast and colon cancers were far more likely to have lived in a high-income neighborhood. The diet of the high-income blocks was not analyzed, but wealthier people are likely to have higher-fat diets. Worldwide, fat intake is strongly associated with wealth, and

Japan is the sole example of a wealthy nation that does not eat a high-fat diet.

All of these epidemiological clues have awakened interest in the effect of diet on cancer, but there's still another reason for the renaissance. The decades spent searching for a cancer-causing virus have not been nearly as fruitful as had been hoped. Viruses are still suspected in some of the rarer forms of cancer, but as far as common cancers of the breast and colon are concerned, no human virus has been found.

Compelled by the correlations between certain cancers and fat intake, scientists have returned to their laboratories to see if modern-day cancer studies will duplicate the findings of the 1940s animal experiments. At the American Health Foundation in New York, where much animal research on fat and cancer has taken place, researchers have found that mice and rats fed high-fat diets develop more breast cancers than animals maintained on low-fat chow. In the case of breast cancer, fat promotes both spontaneous and induced tumors. Spontaneous tumors are those that develop without intentional exposure to a cancer-causing chemical, while induced tumors are those that develop after treatment with a cancer agent.

Mice and rats do not develop humanlike colon tumors spontaneously. For this type of cancer only induced tumors can be studied. When treated with a cancer agent, both mice and rats fed a high-fat diet do develop more colon tumors. These results in animals have been repeated often enough to be labeled "unequivocal." Only a few studies have tested the effects of cholesterol on colon tumors, and some have shown that food cholesterol, too, enhances tumor growth. One study has also reported a worldwide correlation between cholesterol intake and colon cancer. However, because so little work has been done, food cholesterol has been neither absolved nor firmly implicated in cancer. For other cancers linked to fat in epidemiological studies—cancers of the ovary, uterus, prostate, and pancreas—no animal studies have been possible. As a result, the effect of fat in these cancers is speculative.

111

But for breast and colon cancers, the evidence is just short of convincing. The amount of evidence is not overwhelming, but the findings are consistent and the epidemiological correlations very strong. When both animal and population evidence support a relationship, it is rarely taken lightly. At the National Cancer Institute, part of the National Institutes of Health, former director Dr. Arthur Upton explained that a substance that promotes cancer in one animal is more likely than not to do so in other animals. "The totality of experience," said Upton, "shows many more instances where species behave similarly than differently." With the animal and epidemiological evidence that fat promotes breast and colon cancers already accumulated, knowing mechanisms that explain the relationship would make the case convincing.

Much more is known about the likely mechanisms for colon cancer than for breast cancer. For our bodies to digest fat, it must be "emulsified," broken into tiny particles which are kept mixed in the bile. The bile is secreted by the liver and stored in the gall bladder. It's the bile acids, components of the bile, that are suspected in colon cancer. People on high-fat diets have to produce more bile acids than those on a low-fat eating plan. The intestinal bacteria of people on high-fat diets also degrade the bile acids more than is the case for people who eat little fat. The degraded bile acids are suspected as cancer agents, or as cancer promoters. Promoters do not cause cancer themselves, but rather enhance the potency of substances that do, just as a catalyst speeds up a chemical reaction. Researchers at the American Health Foundation have also shown that some of the many bile acids promote cancer in animals. They have also found that colon cancer patients have more bile acids than nonvictims.

The explanation for the relationship between fat and breast cancer has been more elusive, but there are leads. As with colon cancer, fat is suspected not as a direct cause of breast cancer, but as a promoter of the process. Breast cancer, like cancers of the prostate gland and uterus, is a "hormone-dependent" cancer, one that is influenced by the body's hormones. Evidence for the hormone-dependent label comes from research showing that removal of hormone-secreting organs or administration of drugs that counteract hormones has a dramatic effect on the chances of developing these cancers. Removal of a woman's ovaries before her fortieth birthday, for instance, cuts her chances of breast cancer by 75 percent.

Cancer researchers have barely begun to investigate how fat influences a woman's hormone levels. In two studies scientists have found that fat increases levels of the hormone prolactin. One study with South African black women found that substituting a high-fat diet for a low-fat diet caused increases in two hormones—follicle-stimulating hormone and testosterone—and decreases in two other hormones—estradiol and DHEA (dehydroepiandrosterone). These findings must be confirmed in other studies before any conclusions can be made about the effect of diet on hormones. It is also interesting to note that a study of breast cancer patients and their daughters documented higher than average levels of prolactin and estrogen in the daughters' blood. This may help explain why breast cancer runs in families.

One striking finding in cancer research is that some cancers seem most influenced by early life experiences, while others seem to be affected more by late-life changes in life-style. Three kinds of studies, for instance, show that a woman's life-style during her teen years, or during both childhood and adolescence, may have the greatest influence on her risk of breast cancer.

• Women exposed to high levels of radiation during adolescence have a greater risk of breast cancer than women subjected as adults.

• Women who bear a child before age eighteen have less chance of breast cancer than childless women or women who deliver their first child later in life.

• Japanese women who migrated to the United States (as adults) had breast cancer rates closer to the low levels of their native country, though some increase in breast cancer did occur. But

113

children of these women, born in America, have rates of breast cancer closer to their American peers.

Fitting theory around these observations isn't difficult; the breast cells divide and develop during youth and adolescence. It makes sense that the environment during this time could greatly affect the cancer process. If one period of life proves more important than another, however, this does not mean that life-style during the less important period is irrelevant. It would, however, challenge the common argument that only adults should watch their fat intake.

Colon cancer shows a different trend from breast cancer. Japanese men who migrated to the United States quickly experienced rates of colon cancer similar to U.S. men, and female Japanese immigrants also experienced higher colon rates than Japanese natives. Within the U.S. population, scientists have also found some fascinating examples showing that late-life changes in environment seem to affect the odds of colon cancer. People living in the Florida cities of Miami and Tampa have less colon cancer than residents of the Northeast and Midwest. Yet, most of these Florida residents are newcomers who moved there only after retiring from a lifetime of work in the Northeast and Midwest areas of the country. These findings suggest that colon cancer, unlike breast cancer, may be affected equally by all periods of life.

Unlike the heart disease research, which implicates saturated fat as the most harmful form, all fats are suspect for cancers of the breast and colon. A few people insist that only polyunsaturated fats promote cancer, but the evidence does not support this claim.

International breast and colon cancer rates show correlations with the total amount of fat in the diet and with the amount of animal fat. No correlation has been found between vegetable fat—the major source of polyunsaturated fat—and cancers of the breast and colon. Polyunsaturated fats remain suspect in these cancers because of other kinds of evidence, but to blame only polyunsaturated fat when the epidemiological evidence shows correlations only with total fat and animal fat makes little sense. Japan, our favorite comparison country, uses about as much polyunsaturated fat as we do, yet our rates of breast and colon cancers differ tremendously. Colon cancer rates in the United States have remained constant over the last twenty years, despite a 33 percent increase in our use of polyunsaturated fat. Breast cancer, on the other hand, has risen slightly, but because this rise correlates with an increase in both total fat and polyunsaturated fat, interpretation of the findings is difficult.

Though all forms of fat are suspected as cancer promoters, the possibility remains that some fats are more potent than others. In some animal experiments, animals fed only a polyunsaturated fat developed more tumors than animals fed only a saturated fat. But in a recent experiment, Drs. Kenneth Carroll and G. J. Hopkins found no difference in breast tumors among rats fed a diet with 20 percent sunflower oil, and rats fed 3 percent sunflower oil and 17 percent beef tallow or coconut oil (both saturated fats). They concluded that once a minimum level of polyunsaturated fat is present in the diet, all fats promote breast tumors equally. Such a minimal level of polyunsaturated fat would probably be present in most diets containing a mixture of foods.

Heart disease studies where one group of people followed typical American diets while another group followed a diet high in polyunsaturated fat have given mixed results about the effect of different fats on cancer. Taken as a whole, five research studies comparing diets high in polyunsaturated fat to the typical American diet have shown no excess risk of cancer from the polyunsaturated fat. However, one study, the Los Angeles Veterans Study, did show a notably higher cancer rate among men who followed the diet high in polyunsaturated fat. Analysis of the results showed that many of the excess cancer deaths occurred in men who had not adhered well to the cholesterol-lowering diet. For this reason, the scientists who conducted the study felt the evidence was not alarming.

Nonetheless, many heart researchers recommend against diets high in polyunsaturated fat. They know that restriction of saturated fat and cholesterol can usually lower blood cholesterol levels adequately. The Los Angeles study involved a diet with 15 percent of calories from polyunsaturated fat. This is more than any country consumes, and therefore its consequences are unknown. No scientific committee has recommended a diet containing such a high level of polyunsaturated fat for the general public.

Only further research can settle the questions about the different types of fat. In the meantime, current evidence does implicate all forms of fat, and the best approach is to eat less of all forms. As long as questions remain about diets high in polyunsaturated fat, using mono-unsaturated fats to replace some of the saturated fat in the diet is a good approach.

The diet-cancer findings differ from the heart disease findings not just in their emphasis on all fats, but also in the ability to predict risk. Unlike heart disease research, cancer research has not yet identified a simple risk indicator. Science knows that radiation increases the risk of cancer, but lacks a test to show who is most likely to succumb to its ill effects. By contrast, cholesterol-measuring technology, simple tests for blood pressure, and answers to questions such as "Do you smoke?" enable us to predict who is most likely to suffer a heart attack. But for cancer, the message is less flexible; until we can separate high-risk individuals from low-risk, we have to advise everyone concerned about their risk of breast and colon cancers to eat less fat.

Despite some differences between the heart disease and cancer findings, there are similarities. Most obvious is that the fat of meats, dairy products, and egg yolk is implicated in both diseases. "I think it is clear that the American diet is indicted as a cause of coronary artery disease," Dr. Mark Hegsted told the Federal Trade Commission, "and it is pertinent, I think, to point out the same diet is now found in terms of many forms of cancer: breast cancer, cancer of the colon, and others. . . ." For both heart disease and cancer, investing in a lower-fat diet before the disease becomes apparent should yield the best return. And one more similarity that cannot be emphasized enough: both diseases have more than one contributing factor. No one has proposed that diet is the only factor in either heart disease or the cancers linked to fat. In fact, no one has proposed that the fat in food is the only dietary factor that may affect cancer. Research is also concerned with carcinogens that may form when foods are broiled or fried. It's interesting to note that one carcinogen, benzo(a)pyrene, has been found in higher concentrations in high-fat meat than in lean meat.

As with the heart disease research, evidence linking diet to cancer has also raised protests, much of it from scientists long sold on the American diet. "Evidence for a [diet-cancer] relationship is extremely meager. The available evidence is strictly epidemiological in nature and remains to be verified experimentally [in animals]," charged Dr. Gilbert Leveille, who chaired the National Academy of Sciences' Food and Nutrition Board when the Senate Select Committee on Nutrition and Human Needs advocated a lower-fat diet. This argument has become very common. But the first evidence against fat was experimental evidence in animals. And it's been reproduced many times.

Those quick to dismiss the evidence on fat and cancer as "just epidemiological" sometimes use sheerly epidemiological findings themselves. Where breast and colon cancers are low, they say, stomach cancer runs rampant. In other words, if we eat less fat, we'll just get stomach cancer instead. Scientists refer to this situation—one disease high where another is low—as an inverse correlation. Regarding the high rates of stomach cancer where colon and breast cancers are rare, Dr. Pelayo Correa of Louisiana State University Medical Center comments:

> While it is true that this inverse correlation exists in some populations, there are large areas of the world that seem to be free of the epidemic component of both diseases [colon and stomach cancer]. Practically all tropical and subtropical countries with an altitude of around 1,500 meters or less

117

above sea level are free from both epidemics. Recent studies in Brazil have shown that the precursor lesions of both diseases follow independent courses.

In addition, no animal evidence showing that a low-fat diet promotes stomach cancer is available.

Explanations for the high rates of stomach cancer among populations eating low-fat diets have been proposed. Japan has the highest rates of stomach cancer and it's the highly pickled and smoked foods in the Japanese diet that are suspect. Most of the other nations that have high rates of stomach cancer are poor countries, and scientists believe that vitamin C intake may be an important factor. The antioxidant properties of vitamin C may inhibit formation of cancer-causing chemicals in the stomach, and if so, daily access to foods rich in vitamin C would reduce the risk of stomach cancer. But in some poor countries, foods rich in vitamin C are available only seasonally, unlike many affluent countries in which agricultural advancements have resulted in year-round availability of such foods. Regular access to foods rich in vitamin C may even help explain the dramatic decline in our nation's stomach cancer rates during this century.

Defenders of our present diet often argue that we should say nothing of the fat and cancer findings until we can explain the reasons why fat promotes cancer. Knowledge about the likely mechanisms in colon cancer aside, it's important to realize that this standard has not been applied to other problems in nutrition. Several hundred years elapsed between the observation that citrus fruits prevent scurvy and the identification of the substance in fruits that accounts for their preventive effect: vitamin C. No one wanted to keep fruit off the ships in the interim. If research strongly suggests that a lower fat diet would reduce risk of certain cancers, why delay acting until we know exactly why? Dr. Ernest Wynder, president of the American Health Foundation, quotes Immanuel Kant, who said, "It is often necessary to make a decision on the basis of knowledge sufficient for action but insufficient to satisfy the intellect."

Cancers of Affluence?

At the National Cancer Institute, former director Dr. Arthur Upton said he hasn't been waiting for complete intellectual satisfaction. "I've limited my own intake of fat since I was in medical school," said Upton. In one of his final acts before leaving the institute in 1979, he released an official statement advising the public to do the same.

7

A Chicken in Every Pot

Satire was the specialty of the French playwright Molière, regarded by many as the greatest comic author in history. In his last play, *The Imaginary Invalid,* Molière paints the plight of poor Argon, a hypochondriac who blindly follows the insufferable prescriptions of his doctor, Monsieur Purgon. Purgon insists that Argon eat bland food and wine diluted with water. In one of the funniest scenes of the play, Argon's maid, disguised as a doctor, refutes Purgon's advice. "You must drink your wine straight," she tells him, "and to thicken your blood, which is too thin, you must eat good fat beef, good fat pork, good Holland cheese. . . . Your doctor is an ass. I mean to send you one of my own choosing, and I'll come to see you from time to time while I'm in town."

Molière would have a field day with today's nutritionist, who by most accounts, fits the part of a Purgon, who would forbid us all from ever going out with friends for a beer and pizza. Nutritionists, of course, never eat such things, nor do they have time to go out; they're too busy lobbying Congress to bring back Prohibition. The nutritionists, though, want more than alcohol banned; they want whole milk, eggs, cheese, ice cream, salt, sugar, and at least 4,000 other foods outlawed too. Molière would have been joking if he portrayed the nutritionist in this way. Others, it seems, truly believe that the Surgeon General, the Senate Select Committee on Nutrition and Human Needs, and the American Heart Association want us to give up all meat, cheese, eggs, and any semblance of a tasty diet.

"I believe you ought to reopen the hearings and look at all sides of this question before your committee recommends that children stop drinking whole milk and stop eating eggs," Dr. Fred Kummerow, professor at the University of Illinois, wrote to Senator McGovern after his committee's *Dietary Goals* report was published. At a hearing held a few months later, another professor, Dr. Robert Olson, complained that the *Dietary Goals* would reduce the milk and meat groups of the Basic Four to "skim milk . . . poultry, fish, and lentils." Dr. Elizabeth Whelan, director of a conservative scientists' group called the American Council on Science and Health, likened McGovern to the proverbial killjoy. "[Those of us] who read the McGovern report—the one telling us to cut out food additives, sugar, salt, fats, and cholesterol, and anything else that might make us happy—were enraged," she told an audience in 1977.

Admittedly, there were goals for sugar, salt, fat, and cholesterol in the *Dietary Goals* report, but there really was not a goal titled "Stamp Out Happiness." Nor was there any indication that the diet recommended by McGovern's committee, the Surgeon General, or any scientific group involved eliminating meat, cheese, eggs or anything else from the diet. *Cutting back* and *cutting out* have different meanings according to Webster, but not according to the critics of change. For some reason, they insist on portraying advocates of a moderately different diet as fanatics who allow nothing but bread and water. On the contrary, the American Heart Association, perennially accused of X-rating eggs, gives this advice in its cookbook: "Don't forsake the omelet just because it is made with eggs. Make a two-egg omelet with three whites and one yolk. Add a filling. The results: less rich, but scarcely less delicious."

Cutting back on fat by 25 percent—as recommended in the *Dietary Goals* report—still allows a diet with variety and flavor. And as long as you like poultry and fish, you can meet the recommendations on saturated fat without becoming a strict vegetarian who eats no animal products (not that you shouldn't be a vegetarian if you would like to be). But to follow the guidelines, you need good information about the type and amount of fat in food. Unfortunately, facts about the type of fat in food are not readily available. The Food and Drug Administration has lacked authority to require this information on food labels; until recently, the FDA didn't even want such power.

Until Congress gives the FDA this authority, consumers can get little information about the saturated fat and cholesterol content of food. A few companies voluntarily list this information on their food labels; a few more have it and will send it on request. The rest have no information on saturated fat and cholesterol, but usually do know the total fat content of their products. Coping with the information shortage is much easier as a result. Food companies often use shortenings that contain moderate to large amounts of saturated fat; therefore, a product high in total fat content will probably be high in saturated fat. All commercial foods are not high in fat; sometimes only a small amount is used. If fat is one of the *last* ingredients listed, chances are that only a small amount has been used. For the total fat content of both brand name and common foods, see Appendices I and II.

Though the saturated fat and cholesterol content of many brand name foods is unavailable, the U.S. Department of Agriculture does have this information for basic commodities and for some processed foods. Using the USDA's tables, it's possible to rate foods for their effect on blood cholesterol levels. However, it's important to understand that in general the issue is not a matter of the foods that raise blood cholesterol versus the foods that lower it. What matters is a food's effect relative to another food used similarly in the diet. Both chicken fat and beef fat have cholesterol-raising effects, but what's important is that chicken fat has *less* cholesterol-raising effect than beef. The scores that follow show how common foods rate relative to each other. The scores combine the saturated fat, polyunsaturated fat, and cholesterol content of a food into a single score so that you can compare shrimp, a food high in cholesterol but low in saturated fat, to rib roast, which has only moderate amounts of cholesterol but lots of saturated fat. For a low cholesterol level, emphasize the foods with the highest scores, but don't feel that you shouldn't eat any of the low-scoring foods. Remember also that the scores are not the only consideration in choosing foods. No points are added or subtracted for protein, vitamins, minerals, sugar, or fiber—all items to consider in making food choices.

As the scoreboard shows, a cholesterol-lowering diet requires more selectivity than the old Basic Four. A diet that meets the Basic Four's prescriptions with ice cream and whole milk from the milk group, and hot dogs from the meat group is unlikely to keep blood cholesterol low. Still, the Basic Four can be salvaged; mostly, it needs a facelift to remove some of its fat. Each of the four groups does have some items low in fat, saturated fat, and cholesterol. By emphasizing these foods, you can take advantage of the Basic Four's simple approach to nutrient adequacy while still eating a diet that keeps fat, saturated fat, and cholesterol at a moderate level. In the following sections is a "new" Basic Four.

GROUP 1: DAIRY PRODUCTS

For decades, calcium has been the standard for comparing milk products. Nutrition students memorize equivalents for the calcium in a glass of milk: two cups of ice cream or cottage cheese; one cup of yogurt; an ounce and a half of cheddar cheese. The Basic Four recommends two glasses of milk or their equivalent for adults; three to four glasses for children.

But a better Basic Four would consider not just calcium, but fat. Fortunately, low-fat dairy products can provide plenty of calcium, protein, and riboflavin, without the fat and calories of high-fat dairy products.

The Blood Cholesterol Scoreboard

Breakfast Foods

Shredded wheat, most cereals	60
Egg white	60
Wheat germ, 2 Tbsp.	60
Whole wheat bread	60
Buckwheat pancakes, 2-4" cakes	56
English muffin w/ pat marg.	56
Blueberry muffin	50
Bacon, 4 slices	46
Commercial granola*, 1 oz.	46
Bakery donut, plain	38
Pork sausage, 3 links, 2 oz.	34
Egg, 1, whole or yolk	14

*made with coconut oil

Dinner Entrees

	3 oz.	6 oz.
Pink salmon or cod	54	48
Abalone, clams, scallops, flounder, rockfish, haddock, sole, red snapper, trout, whitefish, striped bass, ocean perch, or light tuna	52	44
Oysters	50	40
Anchovies	46	32
Chicken or turkey w/o skin	46	32
Turbot or lobster	44	28
Chicken or turkey w/skin	44	28
Herring	42	24
Sablefish	40	20
Flank steak	36	12
Shrimp	34	8
Ham	32	4
Veal cutlet, ground round or round steak	30	0
Shrimp, fried	26	-8
Pork chop, pork loin, or lamb leg	24	-12
Stewing beef cubes or beef liver	20	-20
Rump roast of beef	18	-24
Sirloin steak	8	-44
Spareribs, untrimmed	6	-48
Lean ground beef	6	-48
Beef rib roast, T-bone steak, or Porterhouse stead	4	−52
Chicken liver, one only		32
three livers		-24
Pizza—¼ of 14" pie		40
½ of 14" pie		20

Side Dishes

Spaghetti or macaroni	60
Tofu, 120 grams	60
Soybeans, ½ cup	60
Tomato soup, 1 cup	60
Macaroni, ½ cup	60
Rice or beans, ½ cup	60
Potato, baked, 1 medium	60
Cottage cheese, 1% fat, ½ cup	58
Shrimp cocktail, 5 pieces	54
Egg noodles, 1 cup	50
Avocado, ½	50
Yogurt, lowfat, 1 cup	48
Cottage cheese, 4% fat, ½ cup	44
French fries, restaurant, 1 bag	40
Yogurt, whole milk, 1 cup	36
Ricotta cheese, part-skim, ½ cup	30
Ricotta cheese, whole milk, ½ cup	10

Snacks and Desserts

Soynuts, 1 oz.	60
Plums, bananas, oranges, grapes, apples, raisins	60
Graham crackers (2), pretzels (3)	60
Cracker Jack	60
Fudgsicle, 3 oz.	60
Angel food cake	60
Fig bars, 4	58
Frozen yogurt, 1 cup	56
Peanuts or Brazil nuts, ⅓ cup	54
Sherbet, 1 cup	48
Candy, milk chocolate, 1 oz.	46
Chocolate pudding, homemade, 4 oz.	46
Ice milk, 1 cup	44
Poundcake or spongecake, 1/16 of cake	44
Apple pie a la mode, ⅛ pie + ½ cup ice cream	24
Ice cream or frozen custard, 1 cup	16
Coconut meat, fresh, 1 piece 2" x 2" x ½"	6

Beverages

Orange or tomato juice, 6 oz.	60
Lemonade or grape drink, 6 oz.	60
Skim milk, 1 cup	58
Lowfat milk, 2% fat, 1 cup	46
Milk, whole, 1 cup	34
Vanilla shake, 11 oz.	30

Q. What's three ounces of meat?

A. Not much. It is equivalent size of: 1 chicken breast half; 2 chicken drumsticks; 2 pcs. light meat turkey 4" x 2"; 4 pcs. dark meat turkey 2" x 2"; 1 veal cutlet 4" x 2"; 1 pc. broiled flounder, 6" x 2"; 1 beef patty, 3" diameter; 2 pcs. round roast, 4" x 2"; 1 pc. sirloin steak, 3" x 3", semi-trimmed; 1 pc. round steak, 4" x 2", untrimmed; 1 beef liver, 7" x 2"; 2 pcs. ham, 4" x 2"; 1½ pork chops semi-trimmed.

Sandwich Fillings

(2 oz. unless specified)

Peanut butter, 2 Tbsp.	58
Pink salmon or tuna, w/mayonnaise	58
Chicken or turkey, no skin, w/mayonnaise	50
Chicken hot dog, 2 oz.	42
Hot dog, regular, one	36
Bologna, 2 slices	32
Mozzarella cheese, part-skim	32
Hard salami	30
Beef hot dog, one	28
Mozzarella cheese, from whole milk	24
Corned beef	18
Swiss or blue cheese	12
Roquefort or brick cheese	10
American cheese	8
Cheddar cheese	4

GROUND RULES

1. The higher the score, the less the food will contribute to a high blood cholesterol level. The worst offenders have the lowest scores.

2. Comparisons are best made only within a category.

3. The scores are relative to each other; they don't represent number of milligrams that a food affects cholesterol levels.

4. Red meat scores represent cooked, semi-trimmed cuts. If more than half the removable fat is trimmed away, the score would improve. If less than half the fat is removed, the score would fall.

5. Adding margarine, mayonnaise, and salad oils does not affect the score significantly, but for other health related reasons it is best not to use too much. *A pat of butter lowers the score 10 points.*

6. Most fruits, vegetables, and grains will have perfect scores. Important exceptions are coconut and avocado.

7. The scores do not reflect any nutritional factors other than a food's contribution to the blood cholesterol. This is an important part of good nutrition, but not the only consideration.

8. For most foods, the scores can be calculated for different serving sizes. To arrive at the score for double the serving size, subtract the current score from 60, then subtract the difference from the current score. Example: Two slices of bologna scores 32; for four slices, subtract 32 from 60; difference: 28. Subtract 28 from 32, to arrive at a score of 4 for four slices.

To half the serving size, add current score to 60 and divide by 2. Example: Two ounces of swiss cheese scores a 12. For one ounce, add 12 to 60, equalling 72, and divide by 2, giving one ounce of swiss cheese a score of 36.

Finding low-fat dairy products isn't always eay in restaurants, but in the supermarket it's no problem at all. To cut back on dairy fat, try some of the following guidelines:

Use low-fat or skim milk in cooking and at the table. In most recipes, skim milk substitutes well for whole milk; non-fat milk powder can be added to thicken it. Buttermilk, which is usually made from skim or 1 percent fat milk, often works well in pancakes and baked goods; evaporated skim milk also gives good results in baking. Most people find that the transition to skim milk is easiest if done gradually; switch from whole to 2 percent lowfat for a month, then try 1 percent low-fat for a month, and finally try skim. If you don't like the taste of skim, low-fat milk, especially the 1 percent low-fat, is an acceptable compromise. (To save money, make your own evaporated skim milk with non-fat milk powder and half as much water as required for making skim milk.)

Use cottage cheese, especially low-fat cottage cheese. Low-cholesterol cookbooks always make good use of this versatile food. When used in casseroles, pancakes, desserts, it tastes good to many who don't like it plain. Regular cottage cheese (4 percent fat by weight) has a little more fat than the low-fat varieties, but ricotta cheese, which is often used interchangeably with cottage cheese, has a still higher fat content.

	Percent of calories from fat	Grams of fat per ½ cup	Calories per ½ cup
Low-fat cottage cheese, 1% fat (by weight)	12	1	82
Low-fat cottage cheese, 2% fat	19	2	101
Cottage cheese, regular, 4% fat	38	5	117
Part-skim ricotta	50	10	171
Whole milk ricotta	66	16	216

Use lowfat yogurt in cooking and on the table. Yogurt can often be substituted for mayonnaise in salad dressings or used alone.

125

Dip ingredients can be added to yogurt instead of to sour cream; yogurt can also replace sour cream on potatoes and vegetables. Adding cornstarch to a small amount of yogurt, then incorporating the mixture into the full batch, keeps yogurt from separating during cooking. Mixed with fruit and juice concentrates, yogurt makes a good milkshake substitute. Always check yogurt labels; some brands are made from whole milk and have twice as much fat as the low-fat varieties.

Use a low-fat coffee creamer. If you drink only one cup of coffee a day, a tablespoon of half-and-half won't add much fat to your diet. But if you drink cup after cup, the fat adds up. Coffee whiteners are usually made with coconut or palm oils, and if used repeatedly, their saturated fat adds up also. Try skim or low-fat milk, evaporated skim milk, or non-fat dry milk in place of cream or coffee whitener.

	Grams of fat per tablespoon	Amount of fat in 6 cups per day (one Tbsp/cup)
Evaporated skim milk	.03	.2
Evaporated whole milk	1.1	7
Non-dairy creamer, liquid	1.5	9
Half-and-half	1.7	10
Coffee (table) cream	2.9	17
Medium cream	3.8	22

Use less hard cheese. "Less cheese" is one of the least popular recommendations for a lower-fat diet, but it's often a necessary change. Most cheeses are made from whole milk, and two ounces—the amount you'd put in a hearty sandwich—contains 14 to 18 grams of fat. (One and a half long slices of Swiss, for instance, weighs two ounces.) Try to use cheese in smaller amounts, and choose part-skim cheeses, such as part-skim mozzarella or Jarlsberg, when possible. The part-skim cheeses average about 9 grams of fat per 2-ounce serving. New low-fat processed cheeses have less fat than the part-skim varieties, but beware of their high sodium content, especially if your blood pressure is above normal.

Whole Milk Cheeses

Blue	Cheddar	Limburger	Port du Salut
Brick	Edam	Monterey	Provolone
Brie	Feta	Some mozzarella	Romano
Camembert	Gouda	Muenster	Roquefort
Caraway	Gruyere	Parmesan	Swiss

Many processed cheeses

Use low-fat frozen dairy products. Ice cream, regrettably, is rich in fat. The standard ice cream has 14 grams per cup; "rich" ice cream has about 24 grams. There are alternatives: frozen low-fat yogurt and sherbet, for instance, have very little fat. Fudge bars and similar products are often made with non-fat or low-fat milk and also have little fat. Ice milk varies in fat content from state to state, but almost always has less fat than ice cream, on the average about half as much. Use ice cream occasionally or in small amounts.

	Grams of fat per cup	Calories
Frozen low-fat yogurt*	2	180
Orange sherbet	2	259
Ice milk*	7	199
Ice cream, regular*	14	257
Ice cream, rich*	24	329

*vanilla flavor

Make your own low-fat cream cheese, sour cream, and whipped topping with low-fat ingredients. For a tasty, low-fat alternative to cream cheese, all you need is a plastic cone for dripping coffee and a coffee filter. Place the filter in the cone, add a cup of yogurt, and let sit over a mug in the refrigerator until the liquid has filtered through—about twelve to twenty-four hours. Instead of sour cream, whip a cup of cottage cheese in a blender with two tablespoons of skim milk and a tablespoon of lemon juice. For a nonfat dessert topping, place a metal bowl and beaters in the freezer until cold. Add one-half cup each of ice water and nonfat milk and whip until the soft-peak stage—about two to three minutes. Add a tablespoon of lemon juice and continue whipping until stiff. Sweeten with sugar and vanilla extract to taste.

GROUP 2: MEAT, POULTRY, FISH, EGGS, LEGUMES AND NUTS

All foods in this group are rich sources of protein, B vitamins, and iron, and the Basic Four recommends two servings per day. But the old Basic Four makes no distinction between three ounces of flounder, with less than a gram of saturated fat, and the same amount of semitrimmed T-bone steak, with 11 grams of saturated fat. And although two small servings from the meat group might not provide too much fat, the old Basic Four gives no warnings about more frequent and larger servings of the high-fat items. To keep the fat from these foods at reasonable levels, try the following guidelines:

Use more poultry. The fat of chickens, turkey, and other fowl is less saturated and more polyunsaturated than the fat of red meats.

Much of the fat in poultry occurs in the skin, and without it chicken and turkey are very lean. Light meat has less fat than dark, but both are lean for foods in this food group. Duck and goose have more fat even if skinned; with the skin, the fat content skyrockets.

Skinning poultry after baking or broiling helps prevent drying, but if the skin is not removed before making soup, it will add fat to the broth. This fat can be easily removed after chilling the soup. Instead of basting poultry with butter, use apple juice or bouillon. Self-basting birds have unnecessary fat—often saturated coconut oil or butter.

Fried chicken has more fat than baked or broiled chicken. The saturated fat content of chicken also increases if it is fried in a saturated shortening, as if often the case in restaurants. Chicken fried in vegetable oil is not high in saturated fat, but has more unsaturated fat and calories than baked or broiled poultry. To cut back on fat when frying chicken use only the breast, the leanest part. You can also make a good imposter for fried chicken in the oven. Season cornflake crumbs with paprika, garlic powder, and a little salt. Skin chicken pieces, then dip each one in low-fat yogurt, then in the crumbs. Bake about 45 minutes at 350°.

	Meat only (light and dark) —grams of fat in 4-ounce serving—	Meat with skin
Chicken, broiler or roaster	7–8	15
Turkey	6	11
Stewing chicken	13	21
Duck	13	32
Goose	14	25

Use more fish. Steamed, broiled, or baked fish is the ideal main course for a cholesterol-lowering dinner. As the Blood Cholesterol Scoreboard shows, fish rates even higher than chicken, because it has less saturated fat. No fish is high in saturated fat, though shrimp is high in cholesterol if eaten by the cup. Still, as the scores show, shrimp is preferable to many red meats, for despite its cholesterol it has virtually no saturated fat. The cholesterol in a shrimp cocktail, by the way, doesn't amount to very much: about 50 mg.

While all fish are low in saturated fat, the total fat content does vary. Some fish have moderate levels of fat, mostly unsaturated, while others have very little of any type. Fish commonly labeled "fatty," however, have no more fat than many cuts of trimmed meat or poultry with skin, so don't worry too much about this distinction.

Lean Fish		Fattier Fish
Abalone	Oysters	Anchovies
Bass	Perch	Herring
Cod	Pollock	Mackerel
Clams	Rockfish	Sablefish

Lean Fish		Fattier Fish
Crab	Scallops	Salmon, red (sockeye) or chinook‡
Flounder	Shrimp*	Sardines
Haddock	Smelt	Whitefish
Halibut	Sole	
Lobster	Tuna (light type	
Mussels	in water)†	

If smothered in cream sauce, butter, or margarine, the lean fish quickly becomes high-fat fish; frying also adds fat. Prepare fish with as little added fat as possible; replace some of the fat with cooking wines. Mix tuna with cottage cheese instead of some or all of the mayonnaise. And try "shake-and-bake" fish instead of fried. Fill a plastic bag with 3 tablespoons of flour, 1½ teaspoon each of powdered thyme and parsley flakes, a crumbled bay leaf, and ¼ teaspoon each of basil, paprika, and salt. Shake well, then dip fish fillets (up to one pound) in the mixture. Bake 25 to 30 minutes at 350°.§

Use more beans, peas, and lentils. The "benevolent bean," as Dr. Ancel Keys called it, ranks high as an alternative to high-fat entrees. All common beans—kidney, pinto, navy, black, and brown—as well as chickpeas, lentils, soybeans, and black-eyed peas merit this name. All provide generous amounts of protein and B vitamins, and with the exception of soybeans, these foods have almost no fat and no cholesterol. Soybeans and tofu have moderate amounts of fat (35 to 40 percent of their calories) but the fat is mostly unsaturated, and they too are welcome on a cholesterol-lowering diet. The fiber in beans may help lower blood cholesterol if you eat large amounts. By the way, beans have no more calories than some other high-protein foods.

*High in cholesterol. Use in small amounts or infrequently.
†Albacore tuna can be very low in fat or fairly high. Domestic albacore is usually high, while imported albacore is usually low. Check the label.
‡Pink or chub salmon has less fat than red (cheaper too).
§Recipe courtesy of the Stanford Heart Disease Prevention Program. Stanford, California 94305.

130

	Calories	Fat (grams)	Protein (grams)
Navy beans, 1 cup	224	1	15
Kidney beans, 1 cup	218	1	14
Lentils, 1 cup	212	trace	16
Chickpeas, 1 cup	289	4	16
Hamburger, very lean, 3 oz.	229	18	15
Cheddar cheese, 2 oz.	226	18	14

Use nuts, seeds, and nut butters in moderation. The fat of most nuts and seeds is unsaturated, and these foods also provide the protein, B vitamins, and iron characteristic of the meat group. If used to replace some of the high-fat meat and dairy products in the diet, nuts and seeds are part of a cholesterol-lowering menu.

Peanut butter is probably the most popular food in this group, and contrary to the rumors, the small amount of hydrogenated vegetable oil added to commercial brands does not increase its saturated fat content very much. Some "natural" peanut butters, though, have no added salt, an advantage over the common varieties.

Nuts and seeds are uniformly high in fat (about 70 to 80 percent of the calories), but the type of fat does vary. Almonds, pecans, and walnuts have the least saturated fat, while Brazil nuts have the most. Walnuts, sunflower, and sesame seeds top the list for polyunsaturated fat.

¼ cup, shelled	Saturated fat (gms)	Polyunsaturated fat (gms)	Total fat (gms)	Calories
Almonds	2	4	19	212
Brazil nuts	5	6	23	229
Cashews	3	1	16	196
Peanuts	4	5	18	210
Peanut butter (2 Tbsp)	3	5	16	188
Pecans	1	4	19	185
Sesame seeds	3	8	20	218
Sunflower Seeds	2	11	17	203
Walnuts (English)	1	10	16	163

131

Use fewer egg yolks. The yolk of a large egg has 250 mg of cholesterol, about 80 percent of the daily limit suggested by some heart disease committees. Two eggs a day is simply incompatible with a cholesterol-lowering diet, unless you eat very little saturated fat. The American Heart Association suggests three yolks per week as a general guide, but most heart researchers agree that children and premenopausal women can use eggs more liberally.

One easy way to watch your egg consumption is to eat the weekly allotment as eggs—scrambled, hard-boiled, etc.—and to find alternatives to eggs used in cooking or baking. Egg white is the first alternative; often, substituting 1½ to 2 whites per whole egg in a recipe works well. If you don't like the results, you can substitute one egg white plus a teaspoon of oil per whole egg; one whole egg and two whites instead of two eggs; or the equivalent in an egg substitute. (An egg separator makes eating fewer yolks much easier.) In baking, a well-beaten banana sometimes works as an egg replacement.

Egg substitutes are mostly egg whites. They have no cholesterol, but different brands vary in fat and calorie content. The sodium content also exceeds that of eggs, though neither eggs nor egg substitutes are high in sodium unless attacked by the salt shaker. The one questionable additive in some egg substitutes is the artificial coloring; some brands use yellow 5, a poorly tested additive that causes hives in a small number of people. (Carotene, another artificial coloring, is safe.) Egg substitutes do work in some recipes where whites alone do not. Recipes calling for separated yolks can sometimes be made successfully with egg substitutes if the number of yolks required is small.

	Cholesterol	Fat (gms)	Calories	Sodium (mgs)
Egg, one large	252	6	82	61
Egg Beaters, ¼ cup (equivalent of 1 egg)	0	0	40	130
Scramblers, ¼ cup (equivalent of 1 egg)	0	3	65	120

Second Nature, ⅙ cup (equivalent of 1 egg)	0	2	40	70

Use less fatty meats; replace them with fish, poultry, and lean red meat. Red meat is a major source of saturated fat in the American diet, not just because meat fat is saturated, but also because we eat so much of it. Beef, lamb, and pork have their good points: protein, vitamins, and minerals, but these benefits come mostly from the muscle of the meat. The fat on the outside and the fat marbled within the muscle is the problem.

Meat is not unwelcome on a cholesterol-lowering diet, but the type and amount eaten greatly affects the fat content of the diet. Trim away as much fat as possible before eating meat. The fat and calorie count can be cut in half by simply removing large chunks of fat on the fatty cuts.

Choose lean meats whenever possible. You don't need a nutritionist to advise you; your eyes can do a good job. Lean meats lack those big white chunks. Rump and round roasts of beef, as well as flank, round, and some sirloin steaks, are usually lean. Leg and loin are the leaner cuts of lamb, and for pork, ham is leanest. If you're avoiding the salt in ham, pork loin and shoulder are the next in line for leanness.

Beef rib roasts, and porterhouse, T-bone, and club steaks are usually high in fat, as are spareribs and other obviously fatty cuts of meat. As fate would have it, the cheapest meat—hamburger—is also rich in fat. Federal law does limit the fat content of ground beef, but the limit is so liberal that hamburger can have as much as 75 percent of its calories from fat. Even "lean" hamburger contains quite a bit of fat, and USDA researchers have found that the fat content of regular and lean hamburger is almost the same after cooking. For very lean ground meat, choose a lean piece of round steak and ask the butcher to grind it. On the average, ground round provides only half as much fat as lean hamburger.

Processed meats such as hot dogs, liverwurst, salami, and bologna are also high in fat and saturated fat. But a few processed meats are sometimes lean—such as ham and some of the new luncheon meats made from turkey. Check the label of turkey products for their fat content; some have only a few grams of fat per serving. Hot-dog addicts can at least switch to the new chicken hot dogs, which have a little less fat and less saturated fat than those made with beef and pork. If eaten in large amounts, bacon also adds much fat to the diet. Canadian bacon is a leaner alternative.

Though many organ meats are low in fat, all are high in cholesterol. The one small liver that comes with a whole chicken contains about 190 mg of cholesterol and can be substituted for an egg. But people watching their cholesterol levels shouldn't make a habit of eating organ meats as a main course, nor of eating paté, which is high in both fat and cholesterol.

Cholesterol in Organ Meats

3 oz., cooked

Liver	
Beef	372 mg
Chicken	634 mg
Heart	
Beef	233 mg
Chicken	196 mg
Kidney, beef, calf, hog, or lamb	683 mg
Sweetbreads	396 mg
Brains, raw	more than 1,700 mg

GROUP 3: FRUITS AND VEGETABLES

Almost all fruits and vegetables are welcome on a cholesterol-lowering diet. All are cholesterol-free, and few have any fat to speak of unless it is added in cooking or at the table.

The exception to this rule is coconut. Coconut is the only vegetable that rivals the saturated fat of high-fat meat and dairy products. Whether fresh or shredded, coconut is little but fat and the fat is highly saturated. Avocadoes are also rich in fat, but the fat is mostly mono-unsaturated. Small amounts are fine, but a whole avocado brings 37 grams of fat. Olives also fall in the mono-unsaturated category. Their fat adds up, however, only if you eat ten or twenty; a few on a salad have negligible fat.

The seal of approval on all other fruits and vegetables also applies to the potato. Potatoes are low in fat, and contrary to their reputation they aren't "fattening." A medium potato has about 100 calories. It also has B vitamins, some vitamin C, potassium, iron, and a small amount of good quality protein. Instead of topping the potato with butter and sour cream, try yogurt seasoned with chives or dill or the sour cream substitute described earlier. It's the high-fat extras on the potato, and not the potato itself, that make the calories add up quickly.

Pectin, a form of fiber found in many fruits and vegetables, may help lower blood cholesterol levels.

GROUP 4: BREADS, GRAINS, AND CEREALS

In some ways, the American diet has improved over the past fifty years, but one of the most disappointing changes has been our steadily falling use of flour and cereal products. Use of wheat products, the most common grain, fell by 50 percent between 1910 and 1976; buckwheat, rye, and corn flour have also lost favor. The American menu today features only one-fourth as much rye, a third as much barley, one-seventh as much corn flour, and less than a tenth as much buckwheat as was eaten in 1910.

Bread, cereals, and pasta—like potatoes—have an undeserved reputation as "just starch." On the contrary, these foods contribute protein, vitamins, and minerals to the diet, and while they have more calories than many vegetables, they are not high-calorie foods. Many of the world's people rely on grains for their calorie and nutrient needs, yet these populations have few dieters in their ranks. The carbohydrate in starchy foods has about the same calorie value as protein—about 4 calories to the gram. Fat has 9 calories to the gram, and it's little wonder that it's the people on high-fat diets who often have the weight problem. For fiber and trace minerals, use whole grain products.

All of the following are good choices for a low-fat diet:

• All loaf breads, bagels, English muffins, pita bread, and most rolls. Croissants are often rich in butter; these, as well as fat added to bread should be minimized.

• All grains, including barley, buckwheat, bulgar, corn, millet, rice, rye, and oatmeal.

• All cereals except granolas made with large amounts of coconut, nuts, and added fat. (Most of the national brands have only moderate amounts of fat, but it is usually coconut oil. Look for a granola made with soybean oil; also avoid overly sugared cereals.)

• All pasta. (Egg noodles have a small amount of cholesterol that macaroni lacks, but are low in fat and permissible for most cholestorol-lowering diets.)

• Any low-fat flour product. Many crackers, grits, pancakes made with skim milk, cornbread, matzoh, and muffins will make the grade. Check the appendix for fat content of common products.

Over the past two decades, low-carbohydrate diets have been promoted as the sure-fire way to lose weight. These diets have contributed to the misconceptions about the calorie content of starchy foods. Low-carbohydrate diets do not limit carbohydrates because of their calorie content. Rather, these diets rely on peculiarities of carbohydrate metabolism to achieve their ends— and the ends are usually not achieved. The body stores a limited amount of carbohydrate, and for each gram stored, it retains 3 to 4 grams of water. When carbohydrate is sharply restricted in the diet, the body burns its own supply, losing the water (and pounds) in the process. The pounds return when normal eating habits resume because the body restores its supplies of carbohyrdrate and water. Long-term use of low-carbohydrate diets may suppress the appetite enough to aid in weight reduction, but the early weight loss results from depletion of the carbohydrate and water stores.

Though the low-carbohydrate diets seem to return under a new name every year, the wave of the future is a higher carbohydrate diet that will help prevent heart disease, and hopefully, common forms of cancer.

MISCELLANEOUS GROUPS: FATS AND OILS; DESSERTS

A supplementary group to the Basic Four includes foods that generally contribute fewer nutrients to the diet than the foods in other groups. Fats, oils, and desserts fall into this supplementary group.

FATS AND OILS

Fats and oils are all high in fat, but the type of fat varies significantly among different varieties. Those watching only the total fat content of their diets may choose to eat butter in small amounts, but when saturated fat is a concern, margarines and vegetable oils are preferable.

Hydrogenation, the process used in making margarines, shortenings, and some vegetable oils, is often misunderstood. Many people believe that the word *hydrogenated* on a food label indicates a product high in saturated fat. This is sometimes, but not always, the case. Hydrogenation is not a black-and-white process that converts all polyunsaturated fat to saturated fat. Many degrees of hydrogenation are possible—producing anything from slight to major changes in the type of fat in food.

Soybean oil is slightly hydrogeneated to modify an unstable form of polyunsaturated fat. This amount of hydrogenation has only small effects on its unsaturated fat content. If a product

137

labeled "partially hydrogenated" is still a liquid oil, the hydrogenation has been slight. A liquid state and substantial hydrogenation are mutually exclusive. Palm and coconut oils, though, are naturally saturated, and hydrogenation increases their saturated fat content from high to higher.

More hydrogenation is necessary to convert liquid oil to margarine than to stabilize soybean oil, but again, the end product is not high in saturated fat. In most margarines, hydrogenation converts some of the polyunsaturated fat to mono-unsaturated fat. Some products are specially designed to retain as much polyunsaturated fat as possible; nonetheless, they do not have as much polyunsaturated fat as the cholesterol-lowering vegetable oils. But the saturated fat content of most retail margarines is remarkably similar. Almost all national brands contain 14 to 18 grams of saturated fat per 100 grams; only the type of unsaturated fat differs from product to product. One hundred grams of butter, on the other hand, has 45 grams of saturated fat.

For shortenings, the story changes. Retail vegetable shortenings contain more saturated fat than margarine. Among the different shortenings, the saturated fat content also varies. If margarine won't work in a recipe, try to use a shortening that has as much polyunsaturated fat as saturated fat. Brands that meet these criteria generally give this information on the label. Shortenings used in commercial baked goods and processed foods are often heavily hydrogenated, resulting in a high saturated fat content if the amount used is large.

Critics of hydrogenation claim that the process creates an unnatural form of fat, known as trans fat or as trans fatty acids. Trans fats are "isomers" of the commonly occurring fats, that is, chemical compounds where the same atoms are present but in a slightly rearranged chemical structure. Trans fats have been charged with contributing to atherosclerosis, but not yet with convincing documentation. A recent review by the Federation of American Societies for Experimental Biology concluded that there is no evidence that trans fats are more harmful than other fats. However, the issue has not been exhaustively researched.

Interestingly, hydrogenated fats are not the only source of trans fats. Trans fats also occur naturally in milk and meat fats, but in smaller quantities than in margarine or shortening.

The charts that follow give type of fat information for oils and margarines. Obviously, all margarines listed are acceptable for cholesterol-lowering diets, as are any of the oils in the cholesterol-lowering and neutral columns. Most bottled salad dressings are made with soybean oil and fall into the polyunsaturated category—unless sour cream or cheese is added. Mayonnaise also falls into the polyunsaturated category. The amount of egg yolk in mayonnaise is small. A tablespoon has 10 mg of cholesterol, allowed even on strict cholesterol-lowering diets.

Cholesterol-lowering oils*	Neutral oils	Cholesterol-raising oils
Safflower	Cottonseed	Coconut
Sunflower	Olive	Palm kernel
Corn	Peanut	Palm
Soybean		
Sesame		
Soybean-cottonseed blend		

Margarines

	Low in Saturated Fat, High in Polyunsaturates	Low in Saturated Fat, High in Mono-unsaturates
Full-fat margarines, 11 grams fat per Tbsp.	Empress corn oil, stick or soft	Autumn
	Empress, regular, soft	Blue Bonnet, stick or soft
	Fleischmann's, stick or soft	Coldbrook, soft
	Mrs. Filbert's corn oil, stick or soft	Empress, regular, stick
	Mrs. Filbert's, regular, soft	Imperial, stick or soft
	Parkay corn oil, soft	Mrs. Filbert's Golden Quarters, stick
	Squeeze Parkay	Parkay corn oil, soft
	Promise, stick or soft	Parkay, regular, soft

*In order of polyunsaturated fat content, starting with most polyunsaturated

	Low in Saturated Fat, High in Polyunsaturates	Low in Saturated Fat, High in Mono-unsaturates
Whipped margarines and "spreads," 7–8 grams fat per Tbsp.	Fleischmann's spread Mrs. Filbert's soft whipped	Blue Bonnet whipped, stick or soft Blue Bonnet spread Imperial whipped Mrs. Filbert's Golden Whipped, sticks Parkay whipped, soft
"Diet" margarines, 6 grams fat per Tbsp.	Fleischmann's diet Imperial diet Parkay diet Weight Watchers diet	Blue Bonnet diet

Note: "Regular" refers to margarines not made from 100% corn oil.

Polyunsaturated fats are recommended to replace some of the saturated fat in our diets, but not all of it. Scientists are cautious about diets very high in polyunsaturated fat, so it's a good idea to replace some saturated fat with mono-unsaturated fat. Olive oil is mono-unsaturated, as is peanut oil. Of the two, olive oil has the better reputation; the Greeks use it generously and have remarkably low heart disease rates. In a few animal studies, peanut oil has produced damage to arteries characteristic of saturated fats. The results are difficult to interpret because peanut oil provided all of the fat in the animals' diet, unlike in our diet, where it provides only a fraction of our fat. The findings are too preliminary to warrant eliminating nuts from your diet, but to play it safe, you may want to emphasize a different oil for cooking and salad dressing. Cottonseed oil is not high in mono-unsaturates; it falls into the "neutral" column because its saturated fat content is high enough to neutralize the effect of its polyunsaturated fat. Many margarines are also high in mono-unsaturated fat.

Whether butter, margarine, or oil, these foods are nothing but fat and should be used only as absolutely necessary for flavor. Lower-fat replacements for margarine, mayonnaise, and regular salad dressings are now available. "Diet" margarines have only half as much fat per tablespoon as regular margarines; "whipped" margarines and "spreads" also have less fat than the regular brands. Diet margarines contain more water than regular margarines, which makes them unsuitable for baking—except in recipes designed for these lower-fat products. The new nonstick cooking sprays in pump-containers are a good alternative for frying; these have little fat, and the ingredients appear safe. Low-calorie salad dressings contain much less fat than standard varieties, and the mayonnaise-like product also called salad dressing has half as much fat as mayonnaise. Fat-free condiments such as jams, jellies, and applesauce offer alternatives to butter and margarine; try glazes, Cumberland sauce, and gravies made from fat-skimmed broth instead of high-fat sauces.

Desserts

Nutritionists have always recommended fruit for dessert. For just as long, people have shown a preference for pies, cakes, and cookies, which often contain large amounts of both fat and sugar. A good compromise between the nutritionist's ideals and the realities of taste is a dessert menu low in saturated fat—or better still, low in all fats. With a little knowledge, the fat content of sweet snacks can be kept to a minimum.

Most commercial pies, pastries, doughnuts, cakes, and cookies cannot be recommended for the cholesterol-conscious. Food manufacturers often use lard, beef fat, or saturated vegetable shortenings in their products. Sometimes the fat is a less saturated soybean shortening, but the consumer rarely knows because food labels feature the never-ending list of and/ors. Nabisco's devil food cakes, for instance, contain "lard and/or partially hydrogenated beef fat, and/or palm oil and/or partially hydrogenated soybean oil." Avoiding all commercial baked goods except those low in total fat is the best way to cope with this problem. A few products are low enough in total fat that the saturated fat content will be reasonable regardless of the kind of fat used.

Cakes: The best cake is angel food—no fat, no cholesterol.

Other cake mixes contain moderate to high amounts of fat in the finished product. Cake mixes are acceptable for a cholesterol-lowering diet only if the dry mix contains little fat, for the product can be prepared with margarine or oil and with a minimum of egg yolk. Note the variation in fat content among different kinds of cakes.

Cake Mixes, prepared as directed	Serving size	Fat per serving	% of calories from fat
Moist & Easy apple-raisin (Duncan Hines)	⅑ cake	4	20
Gingerbread (Betty Crocker)	⅑ cake	6	26
Jell-O Cheesecake (General Foods)	⅛ pie	11	40
Butter recipe layer cake (Pillsbury)	1/12 cake	12	40

The fat content for the same type of cake also varies among manufacturers; check the label for fat content before choosing your brand. Better yet, make your own cakes from scratch. Some homemade recipes take no more time than the cake mixes.

Homemade cakes offer taste and health advantages. At home, you can bake with less saturated fat, less salt, and fewer poorly tested food additives. You can also use whole grain flour, which is more nutritious than the white flour used almost exclusively in commercial mixes.

Recipes calling for chocolate squares can be easily adapted for a cholesterol-lowering diet. Chocolate squares and other products containing cocoa butter do have a fair amount of saturated fat, but cocoa powder has little fat, and a tablespoon of oil added to three tablespoons of cocoa substitutes well for an ounce of baking chocolate. Chocolate syrup that is thin in consistency also has little fat and is permitted on a low-fat diet; such products are usually labeled "chocolate-flavored syrup." Thick chocolate toppings, usually labeled "fudge sauce," have more fat—about 5 grams per two tablespoons as compared to only 1 gram in two tablespoons of the thin syrup. Imitation chocolate chips are usually made with saturated palm kernel oil and should be avoided. Carob candies made with palm oil are also high in saturated fat. Carob powder itself is low in fat.

Greasing pans adds unnecessary fat to cakes. Spraying pans with nonstick cooking spray gives excellent results, and nonstick pans also help.

Most frostings simply add sugar, calories, and 5 to 10 grams of extra fat to a slice of cake. If frosting is a must, the common "seven-minute" frosting made in a double boiler can provide a fat-free icing. A cup of powdered sugar combined with 3 tablespoons skim milk makes enough glaze for a 9″ × 13″ cake or layer cake. Vary the flavor by adding tiny amounts of flavor extracts—vanilla, banana, mint, or orange—to taste.

Cookies and crackers: Cookies usually contain more fat than cakes, more often than not, too much. A few low-fat cookies can be found in the supermarket: raisin-fruit biscuits, fig bars, and gingersnaps. Saltines, zweiback and some other crackers also contain reasonable amounts of fat; choose low-salt versions of these if possible and top them with a low-fat spread. Make your own cookies by using ingredients permitted on cholesterol-lowering diets, and experiment with cutting the fat content of the recipe.

Pies: Commercial pies rarely rate well. Pies harbor fat in their crusts and the pie makers usually use coconut oil, lard, and other saturated fats. Pre-baked pie crusts usually have the same cholesterol-raising ingredients. You can make your own pie crusts using oil; the result is not as flaky but still good.

Graham cracker and oat crusts are also a good alternative to commercial pie crusts, though not all fillings go well with them. For a delicious oat crust, combine 1½ cups oats with four

143

tablespoons each of margarine and sugar. Restricting pie-making to one-crust pies keeps the fat content down. Pumpkin pie and plenty of others don't suffer a bit under the one-crust rule.

Other desserts: Commercial pudding mixes contain only small amounts of fat, and if prepared with skim or 1 percent low-fat milk, are okay for a low-fat diet. Ideally, make your own puddings to avoid the salt and untested additives in the mixes. Plain sugar candies also have little fat and are preferable to high-fat chocolates. If popped with a minimum of fat, popcorn is also a good snack.

Low-fat Snack Foods		High-fat Snack Foods
Angel food cake	Marshmallows	Chocolate
Cracker jack	Mints, plain	Coconut
Fig bars	Pretzels, soft	Doughnuts
Frozen low-fat yogurt	or hard	Frosted cakes, most
Gingersnaps	Raisin-fruit biscuits	Ice cream
Hard candy	Sherbet	Pastries
		Pies
		Potato chips

Most cookies and cakes cannot be categorized because fat content varies among recipes.

SELECTING RECIPES

Discerning the fat content of a recipe is a time-consuming process. Knowing where fat occurs in food isn't enough when you're faced with a combination of ingredients, several contributing fat in significant amounts. There will never be an easy way to determine the fat content at a glance, but a few guidelines can help.

When preparing entrees, choose a recipe requiring no more than ½ tablespoon added fat per serving (2 tablespoons margarine for a typical four-serving recipe). To keep saturated fat at a reasonable level, try not to combine dairy fats with meat. Reserve cheese for recipes made with grains, pasta, or fish, and in these, limit the cheese to at most one cup (unpacked) for four servings.

In baking, try to choose a recipe that meets the following fat limits based on the total amount of flours:

Flour (including oats)	Limit butter or margarine to
1½ cups	¼ cup
2 cups	⅓ cup
2½ cups	½ cup

Many recipes call for more fat than necessary to prepare the dish. Experiment by cutting the butter, margarine, or oil in a recipe by a third; sometimes, even more can be removed. Substitute low-fat, low-cholesterol alternatives for the high-fat meat and dairy products and for some or all of the eggs. Learn to think about quantity; a dusting of cheese or other high-fat ingredient won't add a lot of fat, just as a single egg in a recipe serving six people will not supply large amounts of cholesterol. It's large amounts of high-fat or high-cholesterol ingredients that you should avoid. And next time you buy a cookbook, choose one designed to help you eat less fat.

Nothing makes changing your diet easier than advice from the veterans of the process, and some of these veterans have published their recipes. Cookbooks concerned with fat fall into two categories: those that limit only saturated fat and cholesterol and those limiting all fats. All have some wonderful recipes, but many people will probably find some of the recipes in low-fat cookbooks too bland. Books that do not restrict unsaturated fat have recipes that taste like typical American cooking, but some dishes are too high in unsaturated fat. For a healthy but tasty diet, use some recipes from each kind of book. While you're experimenting, try to use less salt and sugar and more whole grains.

145

Bon Appétit!

Cookbooks with recipes low in saturated fat and cholesterol:

The American Heart Association Cookbook by Ruthe Eshleman and Mary Winston. David McKay, Inc., New York, 1973. This is the basic handbook of low-cholesterol cooking. It features hundreds of recipes, from simple to elegant, and factual information on diet, heart disease, and food composition. Available only in bookstores.

The Jewish Low-Cholesterol Cookbook by Roberta Leviton. Erikkson Press, Middlebury, Vermont, 1978. This book has recipes for traditional Jewish foods as well as for many common dishes. Almost all of the recipes are very simple to follow, and the information sections are good. Available by mail: send $15.95 to Erikkson Press, Battell Building, Middlebury, VT 05753.

Living with High Blood Pressure by Joyce Margie and James Hunt. HLS Press, Bloomfield, New Jersey, 1978. Low-salt, low-sodium cooking is the theme of this book, but the recipes are also designed to reduce saturated fat and cholesterol. The information sections are excellent. Available by mail: send $13.95 to HLS Press, 200 Broadacres Drive, Bloomfield, NJ 07003.

Laurel's Kitchen by Laurel Robertson, Carol Flinders, and Bronwen Godfrey. Nilgiri Press, Petaluma, California, 1976 (hardback); Bantam Books, New York (paperback). Vegetarian cooking is the subject of this book, and many of its recipes are low in saturated fat and cholesterol. It features some unusual-tasting recipes for widening one's horizons beyond the usual American cuisine. The information sections include facts about protein, vitamins, and minerals as well as fats. Available in bookstores.

Cookbooks with recipes low in all fats:

The Alternative Diet Book by William Connor, Sonja Connor, Martha Fry, and Susan Warner. University of Iowa Publications,

Iowa City, Iowa, 1976. This book emphasizes a gradual approach to reducing saturated fat, cholesterol, and total fat in the diet. Many of the recipes are low in all fats, though a few are not. Good information about food composition and heart disease science are included. Available by mail: send $3.95 to University of Iowa Publications, 17 West College Street, Iowa City, IA 52242.

The Live Longer Now Cookbook by Jon Leonard and Elaine Taylor. Grosset and Dunlap, New York, 1977. This is a very low-fat cookbook. The recipes have some added benefits: no salt, sugar, or refined flour. Available in bookstores.

Lean Cuisine by Barbara Gibbons and the editors of Consumer Guide. Publications International, Skokie, Illinois, 1979. Recipes in this creative book are low in fat, but not always low in cholesterol. Substitutions for high-cholesterol ingredients are suggested where needed. Available by mail: send $6.95 to Subscriptions Department, Publications International, 3841 West Oakton Street, Skokie, IL 60076.

8

The Federal Turtle

The wooded countryside of North Karelia, Finland, looks like the perfect place for escaping the curses of industrialization. Snow-covered hills, lakes, and quaint country homes give North Karelia the flavor of a rural retreat where quiet and clean air are the order of the day. But North Karelia's tranquillity is, in a way, only skin deep. For despite its rural beauty and the active life-style of the farmers and lumberjacks who live there, North Karelia has long boasted one of the highest heart disease rates in the world.

About ten years ago, average life expectancy in North Karelia was only sixty-three—an embarrassment for a nation as developed as Finland. Almost everyone had lost a relative to premature heart disease; half of all heart attack victims were younger than sixty-five. "People start to realize that what they see around them is not normal," says Dr. Pekka Puska, professor of medicine at the nearby University of Kuopio. "They begin to say to themselves, 'Something is completely wrong.'"

The people of North Karelia appealed to the Finnish government for help. A community petition, signed by all of Karelia's representatives in the parliament and by top officials of social service organizations, urged government action to stem the appalling toll of heart disease on the Karelian community. That toll was financial as well as emotional: a third of its middle-aged heart attack survivors were collecting disability pay, unable to work, and as many as a third of the county's school children had lost their fathers.

The government responded. National planners came in, surveyed the community, and involved the World Health Organization in planning the most comprehensive self-help health campaign in recent history.

The explanation for North Karelia's misfortune was nothing exotic or earth-shattering. It was, on the contrary, so routine as to be boring. The average adult blood cholesterol level was an astronomical 270 mg—50 mg higher than the U.S. average. About 70 percent of the fat in the high-fat Karelian diet came from dairy products and meat. High blood pressure was common. Smoking was the "only joy" of the hard-working lumbermen and farmers.

With the cooperation of the nearby university, the heart disease prevention program got underway. Program officials went straight to the source of those high cholesterol levels—the local dairy and sausage factory—and asked for cooperation in making lower-fat alternatives available. Low-fat milk became commonplace. A scheme for lowering the saturated fat content of butter—by mixing it with vegetable oil—was developed. The two owners of the sausage factory—themselves heart attack victims—ingeniously lowered the fat content of their sausage by mixing in mushrooms that were growing wild in the beautiful countryside. The government then enlisted the help of the local housewives' organization, the Marthas, in promoting the lower-fat message. High blood pressure screening and treatment was also emphasized, in newspapers and workplaces. An eight-week how-to-stop-smoking course was aired on the local TV station. The aggressive measures began to pay off in no time. Within six years, use of low-fat milk and margarine was up, smoking was down, and high blood pressure treatment flourishing.

It was not the first time that the Finns had set a precedent. In

1968, the Finnish government, along with other Scandinavian countries, became one of the first governments to endorse a diet lower in saturated fat.

Our own government has been the Johnny-come-lately of the diet-heart advocates. What the Scandinavians said in 1968, Uncle Sam did not endorse until 1979. Before the United States took a position on diet and heart disease, government committees in Germany, the Netherlands, and Canada had officially advised diets lower in saturated fat and cholesterol. The governments of Finland and Norway intervened in the food system, making changes in the fat content of foods, while the U.S. officials read medical journals. For twenty years, U.S. government officials were well aware of the case against saturated fat and cholesterol. But they kept quiet, rationalizing their policy of silence by funding research. Billions of dollars were poured into heart research. But hardly a penny went to communicating research results to the American people, and nothing at all was spent toward doing anything like the Finns had done in North Karelia. "All the time I come to the United States I find myself fascinated," said Dr. Pekka Puska, the doctor in charge of North Karelia's massive heart disease cleanup. "You seem to do a very good number of studies, but need to do community work." Puska could not understand why the U.S. government was not more responsive to the needs of its people.

It was in 1959, one year after the New York-based National Health Education Committee had become the first scientific organization to recommend diets lower in saturated fat, that a government coverup began. On December 10, 1959, the Food and Drug Administration adopted its official policy prohibiting claims about the relation of diet to heart disease; in its legalese:

Any claim, whether direct or implied, in the labeling of fats and oils or other fatty substances offered to the general public, that such foods will prevent, mitigate, or cure heart or artery disease, is false and misleading and is considered a misbranding under federal law.

Five years later, the FDA decided that merely labeling a vegetable oil "polyunsaturated" was a violation of the above wisdom, and in May 1964, the agency formally announced plans to prosecute any company that "misbranded" its products with claims of "polyunsaturated." It didn't matter that the products were, in fact, polyunsaturated. The word *polyunsaturated*, even though true, was "false and misleading," according to the FDA, because it implied a benefit to heart health. Even advertising statements such as "Are you concerned about saturated fat?" were pronounced misleading by the FDA! An FDA memo explained that the FDA acted after a consumer survey "indicated that people were misled in believing that these foods (high in polyunsaturates) might reduce blood cholesterol and thus be effective in the treatment or prevention of heart and artery disease." Apparently, the consumers surveyed understood the scientific literature better than the FDA, for by 1964, it was well-established that high cholesterol levels increased the risk of heart disease. Scientists had also shown that saturated fats had a strong cholesterol-raising effect while polyunsaturated fats had some cholesterol-lowering effect. Moreover, the most authoritative heart disease organization in the country, the American Heart Association, had by then urged a shift in the American diet—to less saturated fat, replacing *some* of it with polyunsaturated fat. At stake was much more than the sale of vegetable oils and margarines. Prohibiting use of the word *polyunsaturated* eliminated any interest the food industry would have in making new foods, such as baked goods, with unsaturated instead of saturated fats, since telling the public about the new products' advantage was *verboten*.

The phones started ringing at the FDA only a few days after it announced intent to sue over "polyunsaturated" claims on food labels. The phone calls weren't easy to ignore, for they came from professors at Johns Hopkins, Harvard, and other prestigious institutions—all protesting the FDA's absurdity. A meeting followed where heart scientists urged Dr. Joseph Sadusk, the FDA's medical director, to allow factual labeling about the type of fat in foods. Impressed with their arguments, as well as by a position paper by the American Diabetes Association favoring the same kind of labeling, Sadusk sent a memo to FDA Commissioner George Larrick, proposing that the agency permit fat labeling of foods. Referring to the American Diabetes Association statement in favor of labeling, Sadusk warned, "There is little or no doubt in my mind that the American Heart Association will be prepared to present a statement along similar lines, and I would judge that other professional associations will fall into line with similar statements." Thus, he continued, "It is the opinion of the Bureau of Medicine that it is medically proper to permit manufacturers to label their edible oil products. . . ."

But Sadusk had some competition at the FDA, mainly one of the agency's chief lawyers, Assistant General Counsel William Goodrich. Goodrich did not like the fat labeling idea; he argued that the subject of diet and heart disease was "controversial and unproven" and warned that "Pressing this matter to hearing would involve us in a controversy between the dairy industry and the corn and vegetable oil interests." Instead of telling the public about the type of fat in foods, argued Goodrich, food producers should educate doctors. But he agreed to compromise, if absolutely necessary, and accept labeling of polyunsaturated fat content per 100 grams of food on food labels.

In 1965, the FDA took its first step out of the Dark Ages by proposing that companies be permitted to label the type of fat in their foods. Its proposal was published for comment, and was supported by the American Heart Association, the American Diabetes Association, the American Pharmaceutical Association, and nine of ten doctors and nutritionists who submitted remarks. But a long list of dairies and the American Meat Institute opposed it, and the American Medical Association requested a one-year extension of the comment period. "The only real support for the proposal are a few doctors, three or four drug firms, and three medical societies," wrote FDA regulations worker R. E. Newberry, to his boss. "In sheer numbers, the opponents of the proposal are by far in the lead." Of course, the opponents— mostly vested interests—had been given as much of a vote as the knowledgeable scientists in determining the score. Newberry favored tabling the proposal: in his words, "Perhaps the present answer lies in the opinions of a considerable number of large firms who believe more time is needed to study the problem." The FDA bowed to the "large firms." The proposal was tabled. The FDA had once more killed any incentive for food manufacturers to offer alternatives to foods high in saturated fat.

The American Medical Association reportedly notified FDA in 1967 that it no longer opposed fat labeling. That same year, Dr. Herbert Ley, the new director of the FDA's Bureau of Medicine, followed in the footsteps of his predecessor, Dr. Joseph Sadusk, and formally urged the FDA commissioner to allow fat labeling, which he termed the "only reasonable" course of action. But the agency continued to do nothing. In 1969, exasperated senators on the Senate Select Committee on Nutrition and Human Needs demanded an explanation for the foot-dragging. Ley had been promoted to commissioner by then, and he had changed his mind on the subject. "The scientific correlation between . . . [fat] . . . and arteriosclerosis is an extremely tenuous one," he claimed when pressed to explain FDA's failure to act. ". . . Although there is a great deal of publicity, there is very little fact that clearly links the ingestion of fat in one form or another with heart disease." Forced to account for this sudden reversal of his position, Ley said that on becoming commissioner he had learned of the potential for misleading label claims and therefore now opposed the labeling that he had strongly urged in his lower position as medical director. Were this the real reason, Ley would seem to have been judging his agency too incompetent to devise regulations that would allow for factual label claims while prohibiting misleading ones.

Perhaps the FDA was embarrassed or pressured by this public airing of its bungling. Finally, in 1973, the FDA adopted a regulation that permitted food companies to label the number of grams of saturated and polyunsaturated fat in their products. The program was simply voluntary. To no one's surprise, the dairy and meat industries didn't have any use for it. Margarine and oil producers sometimes took advantage of the provisions. But the FDA wanted to make sure that the public didn't get the idea that they should pay any attention to the labeling. The regulations required that any disclosures of the type of fat or cholesterol content of a food be followed by a disclaimer that reads:

> Information on fat and/or cholesterol content is provided for individuals who, on the advice of a physician, are modifying their total dietary intake of fat and cholesterol.

And while the new FDA regulations finally permitted companies to label the type of fat in their foods, the new fat labeling program was merely part of a larger effort that emphasized vitamins, minerals, and protein much more than the type of fat. Whole milk cartons could tout the high levels of protein, calcium, and riboflavin of their contents without any mention of the saturated fat content, as that was (and still is) optional information. The FDA had devised a way to keep foods rich in saturated fat and cholesterol looking healthful while bowing just enough to the pressures for type-of-fat labeling. And nine years had elapsed between the first recommendation of fat labeling by the FDA's top physician and the initiation of the program.

Labeling of the saturated and unsaturated fat content of foods wasn't the only heart disease issue where the FDA's slowness was incredible. In 1969, at the same hearing where senators challenged FDA Commissioner Ley to explain the agency's slowness in fat labeling, Senator George McGovern suggested that the FDA do something about companies labeling highly saturated coconut oil in their products as "vegetable oil" on the ingredient list. The word *vegetable* implied that the fat was unsaturated, which, as we've seen, is not the case for two forms of vegetable oil—coconut and palm. The FDA was, after all, refusing to allow factual statements about type of fat in foods on the grounds that people might be misled. "Isn't it really more misleading for all practical considerations to permit coconut oil to be labeled 'vegetable oil' than it would be to require listing of such oils and other fats as either saturated or unsaturated?" McGovern asked pointedly. Ley agreed that some change in the coconut oil labeling was in order and promised, "I will do my very best to insure that such a change does occur." That change—a ban on the use of vague words like *vegetable oil* in ingredient listings—took the FDA one year short of a decade to implement. In 1978, new regulations took effect requiring the exact name of the fat to be listed. It was a small victory because the new regulations permitted "and/or labeling." Foods that once contained "vegetable shortening" now contain "one or more of the following: partially hydrogenated soybean oil, and/or partially hydrogenated cottonseed oil, and/or coconut oil, and/or palm oil, and/or peanut oil." Some progress!

As insensitive as the FDA was to the need for fat labeling, its resistance was nothing unusual for a government agency. A few blocks down the street, the U.S. Department of Agriculture likewise did little to incorporate the growing evidence against fat and cholesterol into its food marketing and promotion programs. The USDA had the authority, for instance, to insure that its feeding programs, such as the National School Lunch Program, prohibited high levels of fat, saturated fat, and cholesterol, but the rules of the program had no such limits. Instead, standards for the federally supported school lunches revolved around the Basic Four, and butter and hot dogs remained the order of the day. In 1970, the USDA's own scientists reported that typical school lunches contained even more saturated fat than the average American diet, but USDA decision-makers turned their heads.

The USDA's meat-grading program likewise reflected its devotion to the status quo. Meat grades are assigned mostly on the basis of meat's fat content, with the highest grades reserved for fattiest meat. "We have a major problem as long as the [meat] industry and the USDA push to sell more fat-laden beef from feedlots," heart expert Jeremiah Stamler complained to the Senate Select Committee on Nutrition and Human Needs in 1977. He continued, "The Department of Agriculture is also pushing to help sell more eggs."

He was referring to the Egg Research and Promotion Act, a bill passed by Congress in 1974. The USDA administers the bill, which is "designed to strengthen the egg industry's position in the marketplace, and maintain and expand domestic and foreign markets and uses for eggs . . ." Other commodities, from olives to cotton, have long enjoyed these taxpayer-assisted promotion campaigns. (The farmers pay for the promotion itself, but taxpayers pay the costs of the USDA's administration.) The USDA is only following Congress's orders to administer these promotion programs. But the USDA has the power to approve or disapprove of the farmers' proposed programs. Indications are the USDA rubber-stamps whatever the farmers want to do. About 60 percent of the funds collected for promotion have been used for advertising, while only 16 percent have gone to research.

The USDA's information materials best illustrated its slowness to change its definition of good nutrition. A check on the USDA's nutrition pamphlets in 1977 revealed three booklets about eggs that said nothing about their cholesterol content; a pamphlet about buying milk that did not recommend skim or low-fat milk instead of whole milk; a pamphlet titled *How to Buy Beef Steaks* that praised prime beef as the "ultimate in tenderness, juiciness, and flavor," without mentioning that it's the ultimate in fat content, too; and a pamphlet about cheese that did not acknowledge its high fat content or the problem of saturated fat and heart disease. The toughest-talking of the USDA's materials, *Fats in Food and Diet,* began by assuring readers that "Diet is only one of many factors associated with the development of atherosclerosis and increased risk of coronary heart disease." On the vital question of saturated fat, the pamphlet nonchalantly mentioned: "Sometimes it is suggested that saturated, mono-unsaturated, and polyunsaturated fats should each supply about one-third of the total amount of fat in the diet." How to have such a diet, or just how strongly heart experts recommend it, was never mentioned; rather, the USDA advised that such recommendations have "sparked a great deal of controversy" and concluded with the middle-of-the-road position taken in 1972 by the

American Medical Association and the Food and Nutrition Board of the National Academy of Sciences.

The USDA did go as far as researching the fat issue, quietly, at its Lipid Nutrition Laboratory. It experimented a little bit with the possibilities for producing farm products lower in fat and cholesterol. But it always stopped short of making any meaningful public statement about fat and persisted with plenty of programs that encouraged the status quo. But what could anyone expect from the USDA? Its nutritionists had invented the Basic Four in 1956. Its agriculture experts had helped create high-fat, grain-fed meat. Its officials had pledged their support to beef promotion programs. In short, the USDA had been one driving force behind our saturated fat economy.

While the USDA's protection of the American diet was understandable, though inexcusable, the silence of another government agency—the National Heart, Lung, and Blood Institute—was harder to explain. Though most government agencies are perennially accused of incompetence and bungling, the NHLBI had long distinguished itself with scholarly excellence. Some of the country's top heart disease experts have spent their careers there, and some of the world's most impeccable research has borne its Bethesda, Maryland, postmark. Moreover, NHLBI's scientists, most of them trained in medicine rather than nutrition, were not as prejudiced in favor of the American diet as nutritionists and farm experts.

But the NHLBI's excellence in acquiring knowledge was matched only by its reticence to promote its conclusions. Around 1970, the NHLBI assembled the best minds in heart disease to serve on its Task Force on Arteriosclerosis. The Task Force's 1971 report was a landmark in heart disease history. It endorsed "a statement to the public on risk factors" that concluded: "It . . . would appear prudent for the American people to follow a diet aimed at lowering serum lipid [cholesterol] concentrations. For most individuals, this can be achieved by lowering intake of calories, cholesterol, and saturated fats. . . ." But the NHLBI's top policy-makers rejected the Task Force's position. "It was not felt that the facts supported it," says the current NHLBI director, Dr. Robert Levy, quick to point out that he was not director at the time.

So as of this writing, the NHLBI has declined to give any notable advice about saturated fat and cholesterol to the general public. Its budget for nutrition education has been miniscule, about one-half of one percent of its funds. Its information pamphlets dwell on facts of basic physiology and biochemistry, putting textbook science in lay terms, but doing little to help prevent high blood cholesterol. The NHLBI's war on high blood pressure has remarkably increased the percentage of hypertensives receiving drug treatment. But a high blood-cholesterol prevention or detection program is still being resisted, pending research results expected in the mid-1980s. NHLBI officials say they must have more evidence.

For as long as the NHLBI has refused to adopt the diet recommendations of its own task force (and dozens of other expert panels), it has successfully hidden behind its claim of "insufficient data." At a 1977 Senate hearing on diet and heart disease, NHLBI director Levy explained the institute's position:

In terms of research facts, hard facts, we know enough to treat blood pressure in those who have moderate to severe elevation of blood pressure. We know enough to emphasize cessation of smoking. We know enough to emphasize reduction to ideal body weight. We know enough to encourage exercise.

In terms of the last nutritional issue, the question of lowering cholesterol, the evidence is very suggestive. We feel that because the public has been so confused in the past because of claims and counterclaims, because of bona fide scientific people coming out on both sides of the issue, that in terms of a massive health message, we, in the National Heart, Lung, and Blood Institute, have to get this last piece of evidence, have to get the clinical trials completed, to confirm this.

Lack of evidence is allegedly the problem, but it's obvious that this is actually a red herring. The NHLBI has been applying very different standards to the various risk factors. For inactivity and obesity, an NHLBI review labeling them as "suspected" risk factors has been enough to fulfill the criteria for "hard facts." But for high cholesterol, more powerful evidence implicating it as an "established risk factor" by NHLBI's experts has not been enough. The NHLBI claims it cannot take a position on saturated fat and cholesterol until it has evidence that lowering blood cholesterol levels that have been high for decades is beneficial. But the NHLBI has never proposed that weight control and exercise not be encouraged until studies show positive benefits from losing weight after years of being obese or from exercising after years of a sedentary life-style. Less evidence and less serious evidence has been good enough for obesity and inactivity.

There have been other signs over the years that the stalling at the NHLBI was not simply in the interest of knowledge. The NHLBI director who rejected the Task Force's diet advice in 1971 was Dr. Theodore Cooper. Three years after adopting the NHLBI's ultra-conservative position on saturated fat and cholesterol, Cooper testified at a Federal Trade Commission proceeding against the National Commission on Egg Nutrition. The NCEN, an egg industry group, had been placing ads in newspapers and distributing booklets claiming that cholesterol in egg yolks does not increase the risk of heart disease.

"Dr. Cooper, are you familiar with some of the opinions and studies which are cited in . . . both the booklets and newspaper advertisements?" asked the FTC judge.

"Yes, I am," replied Cooper.

"Now do any of these constitute scientific evidence that eating eggs does not increase the risk of heart disease?" the judge continued.

"No, they do not," replied Cooper.

Cooper, and other scientists who testified on behalf of the FTC, told the judge they believed that increasing egg intake in the American diet would increase the risk of heart disease. By all appearances, he did agree with the conclusions of the NHLBI Task Force regarding the role of diet in heart disease. In 1977, Cooper, who had since become dean at Cornell Medical School, told the Senate Health Subcommittee, "There are many important things that the parents of this country ought to know. . . . First, that their children should not become obese, that they should retain a good weight, that they should have good exercise, that the fat content of their diet should be reduced. . . ." And now that he had left the government, Cooper criticized the NHLBI's record in preventive medicine—the subject of the hearing. "There are many things that the National Institutes of Health could do better," he told the senators.

Cooper, it seemed, did support lower-fat diets and more effort to spread the message—but never seemed willing to say so very loudly while employed by the government. The current director of the NHLBI, Dr. Robert Levy, admits to feeling the same way. Asked what he would tell the American people about saturated fat and cholesterol were he president of the American Heart Association instead of the director of the NHLBI, Levy replied, "Undoubtedly I would be more aggressive in my recommendations than I have been." Levy makes no effort to hide his personal convictions about saturated fat and cholesterol. "The evidence is such that my wife acts on it," he says, revealing that he keeps his own blood cholesterol level "under 200." Science alone cannot explain the NHLBI's inaction.

The NHLBI's silence is particularly notable in light of its congressional mandate. In several pieces of legislation, Congress specifically charged the NHLBI with distributing information about diet and heart disease. A 1972 mandate, for instance, requires the NHLBI to "conduct a program to provide the public and health professionals with health information with regard to cardiovascular . . . disease. . . . Special emphasis shall be placed upon dissemination of information regarding diet." The emphasis on diet was repeated in 1978 legislation directed at the NHLBI.

The NHLBI was reminded from time to time to take its congressional directives more seriously. In a report evaluating the

NHLBI's prevention programs requested by the NHLBI itself, Albert Stunkard, a professor at the University of Pennsylvania, warned that Congress was "deadly serious" about heart disease prevention but concluded that the NHLBI's efforts in preventive medicine were "far from meeting (Congress's) concerns." Stunkard took it upon himself to speculate why the NHLBI was ignoring the law, the findings of its own research, the personal opinions of its upper echelons, and the potential for saving lives. After interviewing dozens of NHLBI employees, congressional aides, and government health officials, he concluded that:

> The problems of the NHLBI in the field of prevention are compounded by the fact that pressures for action from the Congress may be opposed by disinclination for action within the medical profession and even within the Institute. . . . *Concern for prevention could detract from support of basic biomedical research.* [Emphasis added.]

It was another speculation on human nature—the tendency to guard one's own turf. Stunkard believed that the NHLBI stalled on prevention efforts for fear of losing funds for its most prized activity—research. Admitting that the facts were in would mean shifting funds to communications experts who could get the word out. And scientists, who hold research second in importance only to air and water, may perceive preventive efforts as a threat to research opportunities. At least so went Stunkard's thinking, and his insights are shared, at least privately, by many observers, both inside and outside of the NHLBI.

But the strange case of the NHLBI, like heart disease itself, probably has had more than one cause. NHLBI officials have probably feared reprisal from farm interests: lawsuits that would generate bad publicity; and more seriously, lobbying efforts by enraged special interests that might cut into its multi-million-dollar budget. The way to keep the most in the research kitty was to maintain goodwill among as many powerful groups as possible. By not promoting the fat and cholesterol message to the

161

public, the NHLBI has kept the powerful meat, dairy, and egg lobbies happy; by keeping up its commitment to research, it has kept its scientific constituency happy; by pushing drugs to control high blood pressure, it has kept the drug industry happy; and by supplying top-quality information to doctors and science journals, the NHLBI has no doubt eased its conscience about doing something to get the truth out.

NHLBI officials don't deny setting much higher standards for saturated fat and cholesterol than for any other heart disease risk factors. And they acknowledge concerns that the agriculture lobbies could be a risk factor to their own well-being. "I would guess that since there are these interest groups one is going to need harder scientific data to confront them and stay on the scientific floor," acknowledged Director Levy in 1978. And to stay on the scientific floor, the NHLBI needs money from a Congress that has been known to be influenced by the well-oiled wheels of American agriculture. Ironically, the same Congress that has charged the NHLBI with distributing information on diet and heart disease also harasses agencies that make the farm lobbies unhappy.

While the NHLBI devoted itself to keeping quiet about diet, its neighbor, the National Cancer Institute (NCI), was hardly even interested in the possibility that nutrition might influence cancer risk. Throughout most of its history, the lion's share of its money (and it had more than it knew what to do with) has been spent looking for cancer viruses and cures. But thanks to lobbying by the Candlelighters, the parents of children with leukemia, in 1974 Congress created a Diet, Nutrition, and Cancer Program within the Cancer Institute.

From the beginning, the diet program focused mainly on the nutritional problems of cancer patients, certainly a worthwhile use of funds and time. But within the Cancer Institute, at least one person felt that preventive nutrition measures were getting far too little attention. That person was Dr. Gio Gori, the Diet, Nutrition, and Cancer Program's director. Congress had specifically directed the NCI to "collect, analyze, and disseminate information respecting . . . the relationship between diet and cancer." But several years after the diet program was created, NCI was making no effort to distribute literature on the dangers of a high-fat diet, nor advice on how to eat less fat. Its information pamphlets on the various cancers, all given the overly optimistic title, *Progress Against Cancer of the ———, never emphasized a lower-fat diet as a preventive measure. Or even mentioned it, in most cases. As of 1978, NCI pamphlets on cancers of the breast, uterus, and prostate didn't say a word about the research linking fat content of the diet with the disease. Only its pamphlet on colon cancer mentioned diet—one sentence, to be exact—then continued, "extensive research into the relationship between diet and cancer of the colon and rectum is being supported under the National Cancer Program." But Gori, the program director, knew better. Estimates were that the NCI was spending at most one percent of its research dollars in nutrition. One day in 1976, when he had seen enough of the NCI's neglect, Gori took his case to the Senate Select Committee on Nutrition and Human Needs, and requested a Senate hearing for a story that needed to be told.

The July 1976 hearing, "Diet and Cancer," was a great success. Before TV cameras, Gori and other cancer scientists presented animal and human evidence linking diet with cancer. Gori, a key witness, began with these words:

> Mr. Chairman, gentlemen of the Select Committee, nutrition science is coming of age. For years the experimental difficulties in this field have discouraged scientists, who found other subjects more interesting and, apparently, more fitting to human health.

> Indeed, until a few years ago, the role of nutrition in disease was recognized only for certain specific deficiency syndromes, such as beri-beri, scurvy, and rickets, for which rapid nutritional therapies were found. *Until recently, many eyebrows would have been raised by suggesting that an imbalance of*

163

normal dietary components could lead to cancer and cardiovascular diseases.

Today the accumulation of epidemiologic and laboratory evidence in man and animals makes this notion not only possible but certain. [Emphasis added.]

Gori's testimony, not surprisingly, focused on fat as a major promoter of cancer. Impressed with the evidence that he presented (and the lack of attention paid to it), the staff of the Senate Select Committee on Nutrition and Human Needs began work on what was to become one of the most remembered health reports of the century: *Dietary Goals for the United States.* No one knew it at the time, but the *Dietary Goals* report was going to prove one of the most important chapters in the history of government food policy. The chapter began on January 14, 1977, when the Committee released its report.

The *Dietary Goals* were recommended levels of certain elements in food, elements that the National Academy of Sciences' Food and Nutrition Board had ignored. The Food and Nutrition Board sets "recommended dietary allowances" for protein, vitamins, and minerals, but does not address desirable limits for substances such as fat, cholesterol, and salt. The *Dietary Goals* report set such limits, suggesting the following six principles:

- Increase total carbohydrates in the diet.

- Reduce total fat intake by 25 percent.

- Reduce saturated fat by 40 percent.

- Reduce food cholesterol by 40 percent.

- Reduce sugar consumption by 40 percent.

- Reduce salt consumption by a minimum of one-half.

To translate the recommendations into food choices, the report recommended eating less red meat and more fish and poultry;

substituting skim milk for whole; and eating fewer eggs and more fruits, vegetables, and whole grains.

The public welcomed the report. Within two weeks, the Government Printing Office was swamped with 10,000 orders. Some of the country's best-known nutritionists—including columnists Drs. Jean Mayer and Johanna Dwyer—endorsed the report. But in the world of the Basic Four and throughout the cattle, dairy, and egg farms of the United States, the *Dietary Goals* report was considered blasphemy.

No one echoed the old school's meat-milk-and-eggs philosophy better than Dr. George Briggs, nutrition professor at the University of California. In a letter to McGovern, Briggs complained: "Meat, milk, and eggs are among our best foods and we are a healthier nation because we have such good supplies. We need to consume more, not less."

Another University of California professor, Dr. Thomas Jukes, put things more colorfully. "Senator McGovern['s] committee on 'nutrition and human needs' has issued a preposterous report on 'dietary goals' which calls for governmental action to implement the prejudices of its writers. . . . Avast to McGovern and his anonymous bluenoses! 'Tis the season to be jolly! I don't think they know what they're talking about."

Even Dr. Philip Handler, president of the National Academy of Sciences, seemed to be running to the old school's defense. At the 1978 meeting of the American Association for the Advancement of Science, Handler told his audience:

Having more or less successfully managed those diseases occasioned by vitamin deficiencies, endocrine dysfunctions, and bacterial infections, while almost eliminating those virus diseases preventable by immunization, medical research now seeks to address those major degenerative disorders to which humanity remains almost helplessly subject: cancer, cardiovascular disease, multiple sclerosis, arthritis, nephritis, muscular dystrophy, schizophrenia and the rest, including hundreds of genetic disorders. None are necessarily the natural condition of our species. *What must be resisted is the public impulse to address these problems directly before the time is right, to engage in feckless attempts to apply the inapplicable.* [Emphasis added.]

In his laboratory days, Handler, too, had been a vitamin researcher. His work helped conquer pellagra, the niacin deficiency disease.

The old school not only cooked up a cauldron of criticism on the *Dietary Goals,* but refused to grant that the report bore any scientific imprimatur. Four well-qualified scientists served as consultants for the report: Dr. Mark Hegsted, who was then a Harvard professor; Dr. Sheldon Margen of the University of California; Dr. Philip Lee, former assistant secretary for health at HEW; and Dr. Beverly Winikoff, a physician then working at the Rockefeller Foundation. But despite the assistance of these four scientists, the typical complaint held that the report "was written by a bunch of lawyers who don't know anything about nutrition." Dr. Alfred Harper, a University of Wisconsin professor who chaired the National Academy of Sciences' Food and Nutrition Board in 1979, claimed the report was "written by the public relations people on the McGovern Committee Staff." At the American Medical Association, nutrition spokesman Dr. Philip White called the report a "political document." But no one ever explained how the report could work to the political advantage of the Nutrition Committee's chairman, cattle country Senator George McGovern. In South Dakota, McGovern's state, cattle ranching accounts for about two-thirds of farm income. With the meat industry watching his every move, McGovern had called for a diet with less meat. He hadn't done himself any favors.

Though the old-school nutritionists were making enough noise about the *Dietary Goals* to drown out the SST, the backlash of real significance to the senators was the rage of the meat, dairy, and egg interests. Only two weeks after the report was released, there were signs that its advice to "eat less red meat" would be changed

166

to "eat lean meat." At a hearing on heart disease, McGovern asked Dr. Jeremiah Stamler if he would object to such a change in the report, and when Stamler said he would not, McGovern explained:

> I think we ought to do it. One of the problems we're going to bump up against, and we already have, is that the livestock producers are going to start raising cain about this committee telling people to eat less beef.

McGovern had angry cattlemen to cope with, but his colleague, Illinois Senator Charles Percy, had it worse: his state had everything, from pork and beef growers to egg and dairy farmers. And Percy's woes didn't end with his constituents. For him, it was also bad timing. Percy was facing re-election in the following year, and was worried that Phyllis Schlafly would oppose him in the pre-election primary. Schlafly, well known for her opposition to the Equal Rights Amendment, did not run after all, but the specter of a race against her hung heavily on Percy as he listened to the complaints of his furious farmers.

Other senators on the committee also represented farm states: Robert Dole from Kansas and Edward Zorinsky from Nebraska. Richard Schweiker hailed from Pennsylvania, and it, too, had its share of farmers. The pressures on all were intense, but Percy had the most immediate problems, with McGovern a close second. The stage was set for some real tests of political courage.

The battle raged for almost a year, and no one knew during that time where things would stand when the dust had lifted. Much of the war went on behind closed doors, in Senate office buildings, but some of the battles, special hearings granted to the meat and egg industries—were open to the public.

The meat hearing was a sign of the industry's influence. All eight committee senators attended—an unusual sight on Capitol Hill where often only one or two legislators on a committee attend hearings. But though the meat industry was able to obtain the hearing and submit volumes of challenging documents to be

167

published in the hearing record, the hearing wasn't much of a victory for them after all. Things looked good when E. H. Ahrens, a highly regarded professor from Rockefeller University, agreed to testify against the *Dietary Goals,* but this exchange at the hearing didn't help the meat industry's cause:

SENATOR MCGOVERN: If you were sitting where we are, and you read that 92 percent of these doctors surveyed [by Dr. Kaare Norum, Chairman, Institute of Nutrition Research, University of Oslo, Norway] have changed their own dietary patterns, 92 percent of them said they are sufficiently convinced, they are going to reduce fat in their diet, don't you think as members of the Senate we have some obligation to make that information known to the people of this country and to recommend some changes?

DR. AHRENS: I understand perfectly the position you are in, and I sympathize with it. I think if I were in your position I would have reacted the same way.

Witnesses brought in by the egg industry for its special hearing fared no better at presenting arguments to sway the senators. Two scientists—Robert Olson from St. Louis University School of Medicine and Norton Spritz from New York University School of Medicine—appeared on the egg industry's behalf. Olson charged that as far as lowering blood cholesterol level goes, "a positive effect has not been proven."

"In some animals it has been proven," Senator Schweiker informed him.

"You can pick an animal to show anything you want," countered Olson.

A few moments later, the egg industry's other witness, Norton Spritz, interjected that factors other than diet affect cholesterol levels.

"What are some of the factors other than diet?" Schweiker wanted to know.

168

"Some are genetic," replied Spritz.

"That is irrelevant," answered Schweiker. "If we know certain people have genetic propensity to get diseases and we can alter that by diet, why not advise them to change their diets?"

"We have no evidence that if we alter their diet we protect them from heart attack," answered Spritz, who continued, "There is a strong statistical correlation between the number of telephones per capita, for example, and heart attack. Should we tear out the phones? It is the same indirect evidence."

"There is a common factor of affluence," Schweiker immediately explained, as if he were talking scientist-to-scientist. "Affluence determines whether you have phones: wealth determines whether you can afford meat and eggs. Let's not kid ourselves."

By all indications, the senators were not impressed by the arguments of the few professors that the meat and egg industry could muster to protest. But six months had passed since the publication of the *Dietary Goals,* and there were signs that months of political pressure from farm interests were taking their toll on some of the senators.

At the egg hearing, Senator Percy reported on a recent meeting with his Agriculture Advisory Board, a group of farm representatives that he had convened years before to give him political connections with Illinois farm areas. The farmers, said Percy, wanted the problems of alcohol, exercise, and junk food given more attention in a revised report. "It is not known whether fatty acid [fat] and cholesterol cause heart disease; and the dietary goals recommended in the report are not for everyone," Percy said at the hearing. It was a change from the Senator Percy who talked in much more certain tones when the *Dietary Goals* report was first released. In the first edition, Percy wrote:

In addition to acting as a practical guide to promote good eating habits, this report, hopefully, will also serve as a catalyst for government and industry action to facilitate the achievement of the recommended dietary goals. Without government and industry commitment to good nutrition, the American people will continue to eat themselves to poor health.

The Agriculture Advisory Board had given Percy a very hard time at the July 1977 meeting, and there were rumors on Capitol Hill that these normally loyal farm representatives had threatened to campaign against Percy in the upcoming election if he did not withdraw his support of the *Dietary Goals*. (An aide to Percy denied the rumor, but other sources claimed it was true.)

Percy promised the angry group that a revised version of the report would include the disclaimer that he mentioned at the egg hearing—that the words *It is not known whether fatty acid and cholesterol will cause heart disease* would appear in bold type in the food selection section that recommended lower-fat foods. Also to appear would be the reminder "Dietary goals recommended in this report are not for everyone; persons with certain medical problems should consult a physician before changing their eating habits." He also promised that recommendations to eat fewer eggs, less milk fat, and less of other foods rich in saturated fat would be reconsidered, and that the recommendation to "eat less red meat" would be changed to "eat lean red meat."

But when Percy went to Alan Stone, the staff director of the Select Committee, Stone refused to allow the statement that Percy wanted regarding the lack of certainty about fat, cholesterol, and risk of heart disease. Percy tried to have McGovern overrule Stone. McGovern was out of the country at the time, but Percy phoned him in South America in an effort to fulfill his promise to the farm representatives. McGovern, familiar enough with political reality, agreed.

But on his return to the States, McGovern was told flatly by his staff that allowing the "It is not known" statement about diet and heart disease would not only be absurd, but unfair to both the public and the scientists who had worked on the report. After agonizing deliberations, McGovern changed his mind and upheld his staff's decision. He gave his apologies to Percy and decreed that the revised report would not be watered down with unsupportable claims designed solely to appease the farmers.

The second edition of the *Dietary Goals* appeared a few months later, in December 1977. To the amazement of those familiar with the bitter debate and political pressures of the year-long battle, the report was little changed. There were small concessions for all, the result of both scientific and political pressures. For the scientists and industries who complained that obesity is a worse evil than saturated fat, a goal on maintaining normal weight was added. For the egg industry, the committee added a few words stretching the egg recommendation for children and pre-menopausal women. And for the meat industry, the recommendation to "eat less meat" was subtly reworded to read, "Choose meats, poultry, and fish which will reduce saturated fat intake." A chart showed that eating lean cuts and less meat in general was the way to make the goal.

But despite these clarifications, the goals on fat and cholesterol had not been changed. The report remained committed to a diet lower in saturated fat, cholesterol, and total fat. The only real change in commitment was in the form of *who* was willing to stand firmly behind the report. The three forewords to the revised report told the tale. McGovern, chairman of the committee, minced few words. "The purpose of this report is to point out that the eating patterns of this century represent as critical a public health concern as any now before us," he began, commending the recommendations as "based on current scientific evidence." By their silence, Senators Kennedy, Leahy, and Humphrey presumably agreed.

But their other four colleagues were a little weaker in the knees. A foreword from Senator Dole walked a fine line, saying little to indicate either support or lack of it. Dole did describe himself as "pleased that the second edition deletes language from the first edition recommending 'eat less meat' and is not meant to recommend a reduction in intake of nutritious protein foods."

The third foreword, by Senator Percy, reflected his intense political problems. His farm advisers had supplied a variety of

171

nay-saying documents about diet and heart disease. Weaving quotes from these documents among quotes favoring the goals, Percy and an aide wrote an equivocating foreword emphasizing the notion of great controversy.

"I have serious reservations about certain aspects of the report," wrote Percy, noting first a "lack of consensus" on limiting cholesterol in the diet. He went on to advocate the statement that McGovern had refused to put in the report itself. "I feel the American public would be in a better position to exercise freedom of dietary choice if it were stated in bold print on the Goals and Food Selection pages that *the value of dietary change remains controversial and that science cannot at this time insure that an altered diet will provide improved protection from certain killer diseases such as heart disease and cancer.*" [Emphasis from original.] Senators Schweiker and Zorinsky co-signed the foreword. The score was tied: half of the senators stood by the report, while half disassociated themselves, if not completely, at least a little.

The USDA took its cue from the *Dietary Goals* saga. When the report was first issued and the storm still raging, the agency was quiet. For almost two years after the report was published, the USDA maintained that it neither endorsed nor recommended against the *Dietary Goals*. The Department of Health, Education, and Welfare was also silent. But the unwillingness of the Senate Select Committee to change its position despite protests from farm interests was an example to the foot-dragging agencies; if Congress could take a stand, so could they. Even the National Institutes of Health felt a little braver. As an official at the National Heart, Lung, and Blood Institute conceded, the *Dietary Goals* was the first encouragement that NHLBI felt to speak up on saturated fat and cholesterol. "All the pressure in the past has been to keep quiet."

The wheels of change were in motion, aided by a fairly supportive evaluation of the *Dietary Goals* prepared by the conservative American Society of Clinical Nutrition. The FDA and the USDA announced a joint project to evaluate the current

172

nutrition labeling format that emphasizes protein, vitamins, and minerals. The USDA issued a regulation requiring schools to make low-fat milk available as well as a recommendation that schools limit fat, cholesterol, salt, and sugar in school lunches. The USDA also hired Dr. Mark Hegsted, who had worked on the *Dietary Goals* report, to direct its new Human Nutrition Center. In 1980, the USDA and the Department of Health and Human Services (formerly HEW) published their own "dietary guidelines"—ones that resembled a watered-down version of the *Dietary Goals*. "Avoid too much fat, saturated fat and cholesterol" advised the USDA-HHS guidelines. Unfortunately, not all USDA policies conformed to its new position. The agency continued, for example, to buy all the surplus butter that dairy farmers produced. Nonetheless, some change had crept in.

Change was also evident at the National Cancer Institute. According to the NCI, grants for nutrition research increased by 40 percent between 1978 and 1979. But most important, the NCI released a statement in 1979 advising the public to eat less fat. The statement carried qualifications about "incomplete evidence," but nonetheless advised that "a high intake of fat should be avoided." Senator McGovern called it "the beginning of a new era at the National Institutes of Health."

McGovern's committee—which had become the Nutrition Subcommittee of the Senate Agriculture Committee—was waiting for the next big event in that era—similar advice from the National Heart, Lung, and Blood Institute. The National Cancer Institute had acted with far less evidence against fat than the NHLBI already had in its heart disease library. There were signs that the NHLBI might crack just a little. NIH director Dr. Donald Fredrickson, once the laboratory partner of NHLBI director Robert Levy, hinted as much when he told *Science* magazine in 1979:

We've more or less become adjusted to the fact that we probably will never be able to get the ideal proof that we

173

want. . . . The weight of the evidence seems to be strong enough so that we can now direct people toward a kind of set of guidelines.

The same year, a paragraph about diet crept unobtrusively into the NHLBI pamphlet, *Arteriosclerosis*. It was the first NHLBI fact sheet to advise "prudent patterns of diet": less saturated fat, cholesterol, calories, and salt. The NHLBI also joined forces with the Giant Food supermarket chain in co-sponsoring a nutrition education program giving Washington, D.C., shoppers advice about cutting down on fat and cholesterol. But a national effort had not been announced, and the chances that the NHLBI would commit itself to an all-out campaign against high blood cholesterol levels still seemed slim.

The NHLBI's silence about diet and heart disease had always been a powerful force keeping the Basic Four approach to nutrition intact. In 1979, that, too, changed. On July 28, 1979, HEW secretary Joseph Califano and Surgeon General Julius Richmond (both NHLBI's superiors) took the matter into their own hands with the release of *Healthy People: The Surgeon General's Report on Health Promotion and Disease Prevention*. "A good case can be made for the role of high intake of cholesterol and saturated fat, usually of animal origin, in producing high blood cholesterol levels which are associated with atherosclerosis and cardiovascular diseases," said the report. It went a step further, advising Americans to eat less saturated fat and cholesterol. "The weight of the evidence, therefore, now suggests that Americans who have been consuming high fat diets should attempt to reduce serum [blood] cholesterol by changing eating patterns. Moreover, these changes should begin at an early age." The report also recommended that Americans eat less salt and sugar. The government had finally taken a stand.

The long battle for a government position on fat and cholesterol has taught the remarkable truth about health policy: that political pressure often has more effect than the pronouncements of the scientific elite. More than a dozen prestigious scientific bodies had long advocated a diet lower in fat and cholesterol, but Uncle Sam and his regulators never blinked. But when a small Senate committee repeated this unoriginal advice, the Washington bureaucracy started to listen. And to move.

"Tug-of-War Over Diet: Nutrition in America Becomes a Political Hot Potato" read a 1978 headline in *The Washington Post* when the violent reaction to the *Dietary Goals* was going strong. But a year and a half later, the Surgeon General and the USDA had adopted its principles: less fat, less cholesterol, less salt, less sugar had become official government advice. The National Cancer Institute had thrown its hat into the ring, too, advocating less fat and more fruits, vegetables, whole grains and low-fat animal products. By October 1979, *The Washington Post* had changed its headline. "Dietary Goals—Becoming a Matter of National Policy," the replacement proclaimed. But much work remained to get the word out. And the meat, dairy, and egg industries were still determined to keep the message from being heard.

9

The Meat Lobby

The National Archives Building in Washington, D.C., houses not just the nation's political history, but some fascinating items for the food historian. Officials working nearby at the USDA and HEW spent almost twenty years debating before advising the public to eat less fat, yet all the while, a U.S. government poster bearing the same advice was sitting in the Archives Building. The poster, printed in 1917, had this advice for Americans:

> Eat More Corn, Oats and Rye Products—Fish and Poultry—Fruits, Vegetables and Potatoes; Baked, Boiled and Broiled Foods
>
> Eat Less Wheat, Meat, Sugar and Fats

Was it a forgotten predecessor of the *Dietary Goals?*

Not at all. For the advice to eat less meat, sugar, and fats was followed by the words *to save for the Army and our Allies.*

It was a wartime poster, a plea to Americans to change their diets for the sake of their countrymen fighting overseas. Saving meat for the troops was an expression of patriotism. The Armour

176

Company, one of the biggest in the meat-packing business, took great pride in supplying the army during the First World War. In 1919, the company proudly reported to livestock producers about its special contributions to the war effort:

> During 1918, forty percent of the entire Armour output—forty percent of all the Armour activities—were devoted to serving the government. Over a hundred carloads of meat a day, or seventy-five million pounds per month, went forward to the Army. The choicest hogs, the finest beef cattle you raise were reserved by Armour to help feed your boys fighting at the front.

The blue-ribbon label on meat wasn't a phenomenon of wartime, nor did it take research establishing meat as a rich source of protein, vitamins, and minerals to make it one of man's most treasured foods. The importance attached to meat dates back over the centuries, epitomized in literature where the word *meat* often symbolizes a plentiful food supply. Even prayers have reflected the value attached to meat, such as this dinnertime grace dating back to Elizabethan times:

> Gloria deo, sirs, proface
> Attend me now whilst I say grace . . .
> For flesh and fish, of all meates cheefe:
> For cow-heels, chitterlings, tripes and sowse,
> And other meate thats in the house:
> For backs, for breasts, for legges, for loines,
> For pies with raisons, and with proines . . .

And, lest anyone doubt the status meat has held through the ages, consider the plight of Vatel, a master of French cuisine who worked for a relative of Louis XIV. One day in 1671, when the king came to dine, meat ordered for the occasion did not arrive on schedule, and no meat was served to some of the tables. This catastrophe was followed by another: only some of the fish ordered for the next day's lunch was delivered. Vatel considered himself irreparably disgraced, and stabbed himself to death on the spot.

When the last quarter of the twentieth century is recorded in history books, the American Heart Association, Senate Select Committee on Nutrition and Human Needs, and other organizations that have advocated less meat or less meat fat may well look like revolutionaries. In a world that has always reserved highest honors for meat, their recommendations seem radical—especially to the two million cattle ranchers and hog farmers whose livelihood depends upon meat consumption. Cattle and hog farming, of course, are major U.S. industries. In 1978, sale of cattle, calves, and hogs accounted for one-third of the $111 billion in farm receipts.

The *Dietary Goals* report issued by the Senate Select Committee on Nutrition and Human Needs in 1977 sent shock waves through the livestock farms of America. There, in plain English, was a recommendation to eat less meat. The meat farmers could hardly believe their eyes; Congress had never done such a thing. On the contrary, Congress had always viewed meat kindly, as evidenced by the many pieces of legislation designed to protect meat farmers and help the industry grow. The Beef Research and Information Act (Public Law 94-294, passed in 1975), for instance, declares: "It has long been recognized that it is in the public interest to provide an adequate, steady supply of high quality beef and beef products readily available to the consumers of the Nation." The *Dietary Goals* seemed a sharp contradiction, and the meat farmers were incredulous.

But to the scientific observer, it seemed that the meat industry must have been living in a time capsule. The *Dietary Goals* report, as we've seen, was nothing original; more than a dozen scientific bodies had issued the same advice long before the *Goals* were published in 1977. But still the meat producers were flabbergasted. And it wasn't just because the meat producers had neglected to subscribe to the *American Heart Journal, Atherosclerosis Research,* and other medical journals. Their shock resulted not just

178

from ignorance, but from delusion. And the delusion was generated by the people the farmers trusted most: their trade organizations.

On Chicago's Michigan Avenue, the National Live Stock and Meat Board [sic passim] conducts a variety of programs on behalf of meat. The Meat Board funds nutrition research, devises recipes for newspapers, provides materials to schools, and publishes a nutrition newsletter for interested professionals, farmers, and laymen. Livestock producers and meat processors contribute about $4 million each year to fund the Meat Board.

Long ago, when all food was good food and meat was king, the Meat Board's newsletter contained interesting information about all kinds of nutrition issues. For years, board-funded research contributed to nutrition knowledge. Meat Board publications for schools reflected accepted nutrition principles of the times. But in the late 1950s all that started to change. The Meat Board realized that meat was slowly falling off the pedestal in cardiology circles. Not surprisingly, the board wasn't wild about the new state of affairs, but there was a major consolation: neither were some nutrition scientists.

The opposition of some nutritionists to the diet-heart message made possible the strategy that remains in effect at the Meat Board to this very day: namely, to defend meat no matter how massive the evidence against eating too much of it. While the evidence against saturated fat continued to grow, the Meat Board presented a lopsided view of the facts and the strength of the evidence. And the endless excuses offered by nutritionists accustomed to the Basic Four put the imprimatur of science on the Meat Board's rationalizations. At every level—research, education, and information—the Meat Board's activities began to reflect a campaign against the diet-heart message.

The Meat Board says it agrees with the American Heart Association that high blood cholesterol is a risk factor for heart disease. But the board tries to circumvent the cholesterol problem by denying the other part of the equation—that saturated fat raises blood cholesterol levels. During the sixties, when re-

179

searchers conclusively demonstrated the cholesterol-raising effects of saturated fat in human subjects, the Meat Board talked of research with roosters and birds. Classic studies by scientists at the University of Minnesota and at Harvard School of Public Health went unreported, while the Meat Board's newsletter, *Food and Nutrition News,* did find space for a study showing no relation between fat intake and blood cholesterol levels in birds. *Food and Nutrition News* also reported on an experiment showing that protein affects cholesterol levels in roosters more than fat does. "Dietary protein seems to be more pertinent to serum cholesterol levels than dietary fat," commented the newsletter. Reports of experiments with animals more closely related to man—like reports of experiments with humans—were all too rare in the Meat Board's newsletter.

The newsletter also had some problems reporting the facts as they appeared in medical journals. When the *British Journal of Nutrition* reported on the diets and cholesterol levels of Finnish lumberjacks in 1961, the Meat Board's newsletter summarized the findings as follows:

Food intake of lumberjacks in Finland showed calorie intakes averaging 4,573 with 45% derived from fat (60% from milk and butter, 30% from meat and 5% from margarine). *Serum cholesterol levels were within reasonable limits* and no higher than those of other men in the area although only about 7% of the fatty acids were polyunsaturated. [Emphasis added.]

Actually, the authors of the study had said this:

The amount of saturated fatty acids in the diet of the lumberjacks appeared unduly large. . . . *A large proportion of the [blood] cholesterol values was in the range where the risk of atherosclerosis is thought to be increased.* [Emphasis added.]

Most heart researchers would agree that the typical blood cholesterol levels of the men were far from "reasonable." The

180

average levels were 274 for men fifty to fifty-nine; 266 for men forty to forty-nine; 256 for the thirty to thirty-nine-year-olds, and 246 for men only twenty to twenty-nine years of age! The authors of this study did conclude that strenuous exercise might have some cholesterol-lowering effect, but hardly proposed that exercise was enough to counteract the tremendous amount of saturated fat in the diets. So much for getting the facts straight.

The Meat Board has denied the cholesterol-raising effect of saturated fat not only in newsletter reviews of recent research, but also in its leaflets for the layman. Here again, the board ignores direct studies with people showing that saturated fats do raise blood cholesterol. In its pamphlet *Meat and Your Heart,* the group blames population surveys—not direct laboratory evidence—for the bad press on saturated fat:

> There have been a number of studies which tried to correlate dietary factors (types of food rather than amounts consumed) with serum cholesterol levels and/or various types of heart disease. Such studies are responsible for the widely discussed concept that a high consumption of saturated fat may increase serum cholesterol and this in turn may lead to atherosclerosis. Meat fats have generally been the targets for critics urging general diet modification to prevent cholesterol build-up. However, recent studies by W. O. Caster, Ph.D., University of Georgia (*Journal of Nutrition,* June 1975) throw doubt on the validity of these meat criticisms.
>
> Caster's work identified *caproic acid* as the only saturated fatty acid which raises blood and liver cholesterol. *But this is not present in meat or meat fat.* Further studies indicated that *stearic acid,* which frequently is referred to as "the saturated fatty acid of meat fats," *actually lowered blood and liver cholesterol and blood pressure.* [Emphases from original.]

But Caster worked with rats, not people.

Studies with people showed that at least three kinds of saturated fat—lauric acid, myristic acid, and palmitic acid—raise

181

human blood cholesterol levels. Moreover, regardless of what the saturated fat stearic acid might do in a few rat experiments, it has never been shown to lower human blood cholesterol levels— though it may not raise them. And despite the Meat Board's efforts to imply that meat contains mostly stearic acid, red meat fat contains more of the cholesterol-raising palmitic acid than of the possibly neutral stearic acid. "The average blood cholesterol in our people is approximately twice that of people in developing countries," wrote the Meat Board's staff scientist in a 1975 newsletter. "To what extent this is attributable to our diets, which are rich in animal protein foods with their accompanying animal fat and cholesterol, is highly questionable." The Meat Board was fortunate to find two university scientists who supported this reasoning; twice the board's newsletter carried guest articles challenging the well-accepted effect of saturated fat on blood cholesterol.

Aside from fishing for data to absolve saturated fat from cholesterol-raising effects, the Meat Board's other strategy has been to serve as a megaphone for opponents of a diet lower in saturated fat. Around 1960, when the evidence against saturated fat was beginning to accumulate, the Meat Board did allow the issue to be aired in its newsletter. But as the official statements favoring a shift to a diet lower in saturated fat started pouring in, the Meat Board tended to ignore them. Instead of acknowledging the many recommendations as the work of experts, the Meat Board presented articles by the diehards of the Basic Four. The newsletter carried several guest articles damning the *Dietary Goals* and praising the status quo. In addition to presenting a one-sided view of scientific opinion in the newsletter, the board made reprints (100,000 in one case) of papers written by scientists who oppose diet changes, and circulated them to its mailing list. To anyone who relied on the Meat Board for information, it looked like the American Heart Association had a few maniacs running its show while the vast majority of scientists thought the diet-heart connection was hopelessly off-base.

In addition to the arguments in its newsletter and other publications, the Meat Board also circulates its defenses to the media. Some of its news releases reflect opinions, however silly, that it is entitled to. One news release, for instance, charges that the *Dietary Goals* report "may have become a launching pad for a new generation of food faddism and quackery; further, *Dietary Goals* has set much of the food industry off on a righteous search of defenses against patent nonsense."

But other news releases are nothing but sly misrepresentations, such as this one circulated in December 1977:

> . . . Steaks, roasts, and chops are not full of cholesterol, as many have come to believe. . . . Many people are adjusting their diets to control cholesterol by eating less meat and butter, fewer eggs and more poultry and fish. Yet, according to the Meat Board, meat is lower in cholesterol than a number of poultry, fish and seafood items.

Nowhere in the three-page news release did the words *saturated fat* appear, let alone comparisons showing that while meat, poultry, and fish all have comparable amounts of food cholesterol, many cuts of meat have much more saturated fat than poultry or fish. And this wasn't the first time that the Meat Board tried to confuse the public by talking only of food cholesterol and not of saturated fat. The board publishes a shiny card showing the cholesterol content of various foods, with no similar "educational material" showing the saturated fat content of common items.

The Meat Board's record leads to one conclusion: that under no circumstances will it accept the diet-heart recommendations. Its president, David Stroud, says the group seeks "to provoke and stimulate opinion going away from the fashion," and the Meat Board apparently doesn't care if the fashion is the truth. While the board maintains that anything at odds with its position is "unscientific," its leaders essentially admit that they can't be satisfied. When the president, the staff scientist, and the staff nutrition educator were asked what kind of scientific data would convince them that saturated fats—including those in meat—do play a role in heart disease, they gave no answer.

The National Cattlemen's Association, the beef industry's most important representative in Washington, takes its scientific cues from the National Live Stock and Meat Board. The Cattlemen's Association represents the nation's 1.3 million cattle ranchers and cattle feeders. Its monthly newsletter carries the same message to farmers as the Meat Board publications. "Is there a link between the consumption of animal fat and the incidence of heart disease? The supporting evidence is meager at best," begins a typical article in the Cattlemen's *Digest*. "Support for the idea that saturated fat and dietary cholesterol per se are bad . . . appears to be weakening," promised a 1978 issue.

Like the Meat Board, the Cattlemen's Association circulates reprints of articles damning the *Dietary Goals* and similar diet recommendations—without also circulating opinions and experiments that support the advice. News releases, letters to newspapers, and tapes available to radio stations all carry its arguments—including misrepresentations about the effect of saturated fat on blood cholesterol levels.

Both the National Live Stock and Meat Board and the National Cattlemen's Association, along with a few other trade groups, brought their arguments to the Senate Select Committee on Nutrition and Human Needs when the first edition of the *Dietary Goals* was published. They had still another argument: that the committee had not listened to some of the best scientists in the country when formulating the *Goals*. "We had persons we thought were fairly impartial witnesses, starting with the assistant secretary of HEW," Senator Robert Dole responded to that charge. "We have had the director of the National Cancer Institute. We feel that they have some expertise and some qualification. We didn't go out on the street and round up witnesses."

But the National Live Stock and Meat Board maintained that the senators needed to hear still more scientific voices. The board wanted the senators to send the report to a number of scientists for comment. The catch was that the Meat Board wanted to submit a list of hand-picked names. As expected, most of the scientists recommended by the Meat Board were known for their unrelenting faith in the current American diet. The senators agreed to the proposal. Scientists recommended by the Meat Board were asked to evaluate the report, but knowing what the Meat Board had up its sleeve, the Senate Select Committee staff also solicited views from cardiologists and nutritionists not named by the Meat Board. The collected responses were published in an 800-page tome, *Supplemental Views,* that gave the appearance of a fifty-fifty split in opinion about the worthiness of the report.

The meat industry's representatives not only obtained a Senate document for defending meat fat, but also a special Senate hearing. At that hearing, representatives of the meat industry argued that the senators were wrong to support the proposed diet changes when some scientists did not agree. Senator Robert Dole of Kansas reminded them that many times Congress had sided *with* the meat industry when other voices were begging it not to. When the shoe was on the other foot, when Congress was acting on the meat industry's behalf, the meat producers had not objected to action in the face of disagreement. Dole recalled some of these occasions.

I remember the Beef Research and Information Act. There was opposition to that act, but it passed the Congress and it will be helpful to your industry, if you can get the referendum passed.

I think of the time we spent expanding animal health research, through appropriations and expanded assistance to veterinary schools. I am reminded of the Parker bill to assure prompt payment to the cattlemen. There wasn't unanimous opinion on that either, but there are some of us on this jury that thought it was necessary to help the industry.

I remember working on Federal meat inspection legislation to preserve State meat inspectors. I remember the research program to help the livestock industry, which was very controversial. It was compared to Lockheed, another bailout program, but here again we felt it was needed by the industry.

I recall testifying at the Public Works Committee so we could find the source points of pollution, which we think is critical to ycur industry.

I remember last year, in September and October, in the heat of other business, discussing with the then President, the Meat Import Quota Act, because I thought that was helpful to your industry.

Many times I have urged, as have other Senators, the Secretaries of Agriculture and Defense to increase appropriations for advance purchase of meat to help a sagging market. I recall fighting harassment from OSHA and EPA on behalf of the cattlemen and supporting legislation to label imported meat the same as domestic meat, and calling on the Department of Agriculture and the State Department to break down tariffs and discriminatory fees against our beef, so we could export some to Japan and other countries.

I say that not as a litany of what happened, but to get the proper perspective in this hearing.

And after reminding livestock producers that Congress had hardly turned a deaf ear to its every request, Dole gave his own reaction to the way meat interests had handled their opposition to the *Dietary Goals:*

I have found that once there is even a hint of disagreement [from Congress] with your industry, there is a violent reaction. Some of it was totally inaccurate in my State, and just off the top of the hat.

We resent things like that, just as you do. It seems to us that if we have to take an oath to always support the cattle

186

industry—or any other special interest group—to stay in Congress, then I don't want to be in the Congress in that event.

But when the Senate Select Committee published the second edition of the *Dietary Goals* nine months later, Dole once more supported the meat industry's cause. "I am pleased that the second edition deletes language from the first edition recommending 'eat less meat' and is not meant to recommend a reduction in intake of nutritious protein foods," he wrote in his foreword.

This change in wording—from "decrease consumption of meat and increase consumption of poultry and fish" to "decrease consumption of animal fat, and choose meats, poultry, and fish which will reduce saturated fat intake" was hardly enough to please the Meat Board or the National Cattlemen's Association. The groups still maintained that the report was hogwash, and they continued to assure their constituents that the evidence against saturated fat was slim. And though the meat industry representatives felt they had lost their battle with McGovern's committee, they won a major round in Congress by defeating the National Consumer Nutrition Information Act, a bill that would have allocated $10 million for nutrition education programs. The bill was approved by the Subcommittee on Domestic Marketing, Consumer Relations, and Nutrition, only to be killed by the full House Agriculture Committee. The National Cattlemen's Association had written to Congressman Thomas Foley, chairman of the House Agriculture Committee, to oppose the bill. "Much misleading and erroneous information, particularly about the value of beef in the diet, is being disseminated to the public by various segments of our society, including the federal government," wrote the group. "Such information is often based on preliminary findings, supposition, inconclusive evidence or political considerations." After the Agriculture Committee killed the bill, *Advertising Age,* a trade journal, reported that meat and egg interests were responsible. "The commodity groups were said to be edgy about how such a nutrition education campaign would handle the cholesterol issue," said the journal.

Looking for still other ways to combat criticism of meat fat, the National Cattlemen's Association also revived the Beef Research and Information Act. The bill, passed by Congress in 1976, authorized the USDA to administer a beef promotion program—if two-thirds of the beef producers favored one. The farmers contribute a fraction of their income for such a program, though taxpayers fund the cost of USDA's administration. But after the bill passed Congress, fewer than two-thirds of the farmers voted to go ahead with the program. Proponents of the bill went back to Capitol Hill and convinced Congress to change the rules of the game. Congress agreed, amending the bill to require only a majority of livestock producers—not two-thirds— to vote "yes" in order to make the program a reality. But even on the second try, less than half the farmers voted for the new promotion program. Weren't the National Live Stock and Meat Board and the National Cattlemen's Association doing a good enough job of creating confusion?

Some of the smaller trade associations have also tried to quiet recommendations to eat less meat fat. When the National Heart, Lung, and Blood Institute co-sponsored a nutrition education program with the Giant Food supermarket chain, the North Central Montana Stockgrowers Association sent this resolution to Montana Senator Max Baucus:

> Whereas a branch of the United States Department of Health, Education and Welfare, known as the National Heart, Blood and Lung Institute [sic], is operating a pilot program called "Foods for Health"; which advertises against beef and fats. And whereas beef has never been found to be harmful to people.
>
> Let it be resolved North Central Montana Stockgrowers Assn., Inc., demands this program be stopped to save our

tax money so people can continue to have a healthy diet of beef.

Baucus sent the resolution to NHLBI's boss, Health, Education and Welfare Secretary Joseph Califano. "I would appreciate your reviewing the concerns expressed by the [North Central Montana Stockgrowers] Association," wrote Baucus. "As you know, Montana's beef industry is large and I would be concerned about any program which might threaten thousands of people engaged in the livestock occupation."

To be sure, there is no shortage of pressure from the meat industry. And it's only one-third of the story.

10

The Dairy Lobby

"Nutrition: Stepchild of the Medical Sciences," read the headline on a 1979 editorial in *The Washington Post,* and most would agree with its argument that nutrition has too long been a low priority in medical research. "The subject does not have the glamour it had in the days of the discovery of the vitamins," Rockefeller University professor E. H. Ahrens told senators at a hearing in 1977. "It has fallen on hard times."

But senior members of the nutrition profession remember well the vitamin discovery era—a period that began in 1913, with the discovery of vitamin A, and ended in 1948 when the last vitamin, B_{12}, was discovered. And in 1979, nutritionists commemorated the centennial of the birth of the man who started it all: a scientific pioneer named Elmer McCollum. McCollum discovered not only the first vitamin, vitamin A, but also vitamin D in 1922. The techniques he developed in his own experiments became classic methods used by other investigators studying vitamin needs. "He changed our understanding of nutrition in much the same way as Albert Einstein revolutionized the study of the universe," commented nutritionists Drs. Jean Mayer and Johanna Dwyer.

McCollum did more than stay in his laboratory searching for

vitamins. He wrote five editions of a widely used textbook, several popular books, and dozens of articles for magazines. During World War I, he served on President Hoover's U.S. Food Administration, touring the country on its behalf to give advice on meeting nutrient needs with what foods were available. He worked closely with professional organizations and farmers. His active career inspired dozens of scientists around him, and because nutrition bears so directly on health, his work also drew attention from policymakers.

It was in the winter of 1922 that nutrition scientists, responding to a call from President Warren Harding, came to the White House for a conference on food and agriculture. Of special concern was a new dairy product made by blending evaporated skim milk with vegetable oil—a product known by the odd-sounding name "filled milk." Very little was known about vitamins at the time; scientists had good evidence of only four vitamins in food. But thanks to Elmer McCollum, the scientists did know that milk fat contained vitamin A, and that vegetable fat did not. In McCollum's experiments, rats fed olive oil grew poorly and developed eye diseases while rats fed milk fat grew well and were free of eye disorders. The idea of replacing the naturally occurring fat in milk with vegetable oil made the conference scientists see red. Using language uncharacteristic of their profession, they called filled milk "a growing menace" to public health and urged state and national legislatures to ban it.

The following year, the filled milk issue went to Capitol Hill, where Congress, acting on the advice of the scientists, took the strongest action possible. The 1923 Filled Milk Act prohibited shipment of filled milk across state lines. Congress did not have the power to stop the sale of filled milk within the state where it was manufactured, but some states solved that problem with their own laws outlawing the product. The laws reflected scientific thought of the time: that milk fat was a major source of nutrients that no other food could provide.

No one was more convinced of milk's importance than Elmer McCollum, and by milk, he meant whole milk. "The liberal consumers of milk and its products are the only peoples in the world who have achieved a great mastery over the forces of nature, and who have excelled in every line of mental activity," he told an audience in 1918. "They are the only peoples who have devised such political systems as offer good opportunities for the individual of low birth to develop his powers." McCollum coined the term *protective foods,* to describe foods rich in vitamin A. By his standard, butter, whole milk, eggs, and leafy green vegetables were protective foods, a designation that some nutritionists still use today.

McCollum's work also convinced others that milk fat was as good as gold. When the New York State legislature was considering action against filled milk, Dr. William Geis, chairman of the biochemistry department of Columbia University College of Physicians and Surgeons, urged a ban. "I am in favor of prohibiting the manufacture and sale of filled milk," said Geis. "There is no economic necessity in our country for this imitation and debasement of pure evaporated milk. There is a biological function of butterfat [milk fat] which cannot be supplied by any vegetable fat in combination with skimmed milk."

Though only a few vitamins were known to exist at the time, scientists believed that quite a few others remained to be found. There was speculation at the time that not just the vitamin A, but all of the vitamins in milk occurred in the fat. In proposing legislation to ban filled milk, the Senate Committee on Agriculture and Forestry revealed the esteem accorded to milk fat:

In recent years scientists have discovered food elements known as "vitamines" which are highly essential to the growth and well-being of the human body. . . . Our chief source of the vitamines is milk, and *the vitamines are found almost wholly in the butterfat of the milk.* . . . It is a curious fact that all vegetable oils and fats are wholly lacking in vitamines. . . . It is therefore all the more necessary that we supply the vitamines in the milk. Milk is one chief food of

192

the nation and no adulteration of it or substitution for it should be permitted. [Emphasis added.]

The committee's report went on to praise the dairy industry. "Dairying represents the highest point reached in the farm economy," said the report. "Wherever dairying is extensively practiced, the entire community reflects its benefits."

With nutritionists such as Elmer McCollum advocating dairy products, dairy farming did become extensively practiced. Congress, wanting to protect a growing constituency—the dairy farmers—eventually adopted legislation far more important to dairymen than the Filled Milk Act. In 1949, the government adopted its program of price supports for dairy farmers. The price supports guarantee farmers a minimum return for all the milk they produce.

The government can achieve price supports in several ways; it can pay farmers directly or it can purchase leftover farm products. In 1949, when the price support program began, the second option was chosen. The USDA agreed to set a minimum price for milk each year, and to buy any milk that farmers couldn't sell to the public for at least the minimum price. The leftovers, delivered to the USDA in the form of butter, American cheese, and nonfat dry milk, became USDA property to be allocated as the government saw fit.

It was only consistent with the nutritional wisdom of the time for the USDA to distribute the dairy surplus to schools, the military, and prisons. "Milk is our greatest protective food and its use must be increased rather than diminished. The liberal use of milk has made us what we are," Elmer McCollum would say. Achieving price supports through distribution of excess dairy products to school lunchrooms and military mess halls contributed something for everyone: the farmers received compensation for their work and the kids and servicemen got protein, calcium, and vitamins from the cheese and milk and vitamin A from the butter.

193

Elmer McCollum had two more ideas to help the farmers and public alike. He urged the farmers to fund nutrition education programs—predicting that such educational campaigns would help the public choose a healthier diet while helping the farmers sell more of their products. In 1915, the dairy farmers took his advice and founded the National Dairy Council to educate the public about good nutrition. Nutritionists and teachers applauded the idea, appreciating the educational materials provided by the Dairy Council. Everyone realized that the Dairy Council had a vested interest in urging children to drink milk, but their parents and teachers wanted much the same, so no one objected to making the Dairy Council the nation's de facto nutrition educator.

But McCollum wanted the farmers to fund scientific research as well as educational campaigns. "Research has supplied and will continue to supply 'selling points' for old products," he said in a 1933 speech entitled "The Business Value of Research." Nutrition science has grown around the benefits ("selling points") in food, and McCollum believed that continued research would only provide evidence of still unidentified benefits. In McCollum's view, such research would also help both the public and the farmers.

"We find perhaps no better example of the value of scientific research to industry in monetary returns, in building up the magnitude of the industry, in making profitable agriculture, and in improving the character of the human diet, than in the application of science to the dairy industry," said McCollum in that 1933 speech. The dairy farmers, who held McCollum their hero, decided once more to take his advice. In 1941, the dairy farmers expanded the National Dairy Council's agenda to include funding of university research. It was a hefty investment, but the farmers were confident, as was McCollum, that the research money would pay off in increased sales. Scientists, of course, appreciated the research funds.

Research funded by the Dairy Council did contribute important information about the nutritional value of milk—just as

McCollum had predicted. But midway into the 1950s, the plan went haywire. A study funded by the National Dairy Council became one of the first to reveal not just the "selling points" for dairy products, but the nonselling points. Three University of Minnesota researchers who were to become leaders in heart disease research—Drs. Ancel Keys, Joseph Anderson, and Francisco Grande—reported in 1957 that butter had more cholesterol-raising effect than any of the vegetable or fish oils studied. In their study group of eighteen men, a diet containing 100 grams of butter per day caused cholesterol levels 42 mg higher than a diet with an equal amount of cottonseed oil. The idea that nutrition research would uncover only "good things" was on its way out. Continued research confirmed findings that butter has more cholesterol-raising effect than most fats, and that cholesterol levels strongly influence chances of heart disease. McCollum had not anticipated that nutrition scientists would discover ill effects of food components, putting agriculture on the defensive. His description of whole milk and egg yolk as "protective foods" (for their vitamin A content) became tarnished by findings that the saturated fat and cholesterol in milk fat and egg yolk have cholesterol-raising effects.

Other beliefs dating back to the time of McCollum's groundbreaking research on vitamins have also changed. The 1923 Senate report on filled milk, for instance, had said: "Our chief source of the vitamines is milk, and the vitamines are found almost wholly in the butterfat of the milk. . . . It is a curious fact that all vegetable oils and fats are wholly lacking in vitamines." But later research showed that foods other than milk also contain generous amounts of vitamins. Moreover, the B vitamins in milk—not to mention the protein and calcium—were not found in the fat, but in the fat-free portion that remains when milk is skimmed. (The addition of vitamin A to skim milk—now federal law—makes skim milk as nutritious as whole, with less fat and fewer calories.) And contrary to 1923 beliefs, vegetable fats proved to contain some vitamins after all—namely, vitamin E. Researchers also found most vegetable oils rich in the essential fat,

195

linoleic acid. Most importantly, though, milk fat was found to be rich in the saturated fats that raise blood cholesterol levels. This last finding, more than any other, brought science full circle during the twentieth century: from treasuring milk fat to suspecting it.

Policy, of course, must have changed with the new science. Congress must have overturned the Filled Milk Act on learning that milk fat was not an essential source of nutrients, as once believed. The USDA must have found a different way to administer dairy price supports so that school lunchrooms and military mess halls would not remain dumping grounds for unwanted butter, with its saturated fat. The health community must have replaced the National Dairy Council's educational materials that emphasize high-fat dairy products with up-to-date materials addressing the problems of diets high in fat. Of course. But sadly, this is hardly what has happened. *Despite the wealth of knowledge about diet and heart disease, policy has remained firmly rooted in the beliefs of the 1920s.*

Filled milk, for instance, remains illegal in about twenty states—and was illegal nationwide until a federal court declared the law unconstitutional in 1972. The USDA still achieves price supports through purchases of butter, cheese, and dry milk. Though some of the nonfat milk is donated to other nations, all of the butter and cheese is channeled into school lunchrooms, military mess halls, welfare programs, and prisons. During the 1976–77 farm year, for example, the USDA dropped 86 million pounds of butter at the doorsteps of institutional feeding programs. The National Dairy Council remains the biggest supplier of nutrition education materials for schools—even though its materials still plug high-fat dairy products and give short shrift to low-fat varieties. The failure of policy to move forward with the times can be attributed to two forces working in concert: outdated but lingering ideas about high-fat dairy products; and a powerful dairy industry still valuing milk fat the way Elmer McCollum did. The dairy farmers don't value milk fat simply for its vitamin A content, but also for its cash value.

Ironically, the man responsible for the high cash value of milk fat was a close friend of Elmer McCollum. He was Dr. Stephen Babcock, a scientist who was already working at the University of Wisconsin College of Agriculture when McCollum joined the faculty in 1907. Babcock invented a simple but precise test for the fat content of milk, and his test became the basis for paying farmers for their milk. Pricing milk by its fat content made sense in 1890, when Babcock perfected his method, because at that time much milk was sold for making butter and cream—both mostly fat. The fat-pricing system also helped solve two of the earliest forms of dairy corruption: illegal watering and skimming of cow's milk to make a fast buck. Before milk was priced by its fat content, adding water would increase the volume of a given amount of milk, while skimming would make two products out of one. Babcock's fat test helped put an end to that.

But paying farmers on the basis of the fat in the animal's milk made milk fat the most valued part of the milk. This policy encouraged farmers to breed cows that produce high-fat milk and, conversely, to slaughter cows producing low-fat milk and sell their meat as hamburger. Unlike the Filled Milk Act, the milk-pricing system was not adopted with perceived health benefits in mind. Nonetheless, the system originated when health scientists had no reason to believe that any harm would result. Unfortunately, in most parts of the country, the fat-pricing system remains in effect; in a few states, fat content is simply one of several factors involved in pricing milk from the farm. While medical journals publish articles about the problems of high-fat diets, dairy magazines contain articles on how to boost the fat content of the cow's milk. (If all else fails, of course, the cow goes to the slaughterhouse.)

Other dairy policies adopted before scientists had reason to object have also survived the accumulation of evidence that should have forced updating of the lawbooks.

At the national level, the Food and Drug Administration sets standards for the milk fat content of various dairy foods. Because milk fat is the most valuable portion of the milk, states acting in the interest of dairy farmers sometimes go further than the FDA and require more fat than the federal standard. In such states, products containing the minimum level set by the FDA cannot be sold; they must meet the higher state standard. In some cases, the higher state standards add only slight amounts of fat to dairy products. The FDA, for instance, requires that whole milk contain at least 3.25 percent fat by weight—about half the calories in the milk. Eleven states require higher fat levels—often about 3.5 percent fat by weight. This additional amount adds only about half a gram of fat to a glass of whole milk.

In other cases, however, the higher state standards add significant amounts of fat. The FDA allows low-fat milk to contain as little as 0.5 percent fat by weight, but California, North Dakota, and Washington require at least 1.9 percent—which translates into three more grams of fat per glass. The FDA also permits ice milk with as little as 2 percent fat by weight; but Arizona, Louisiana, and South Carolina require a minimum of 4 percent fat—adding about 3 grams of fat per cup. Arkansas, Massachusetts, South Carolina, and Utah also allow higher levels of fat in ice milk than the federal standard. The FDA sets a maximum level of 7 percent fat by weight for ice milk, but these four states allow up to 10 percent fat by weight. The difference between the FDA's maximum and the 10 percent level amounts to about 4 grams of fat per cup. But South Dakota and Maine have the most incredible pro-milk-fat laws. When the USDA surveyed state dairy laws in 1977, low-fat cottage cheese was illegal in these two states.

State laws also act on behalf of milk fat by restricting the sale of dairy products made with vegetable oil in place of milk fat. It's not just filled milk that can't be sold; about two dozen states ban mellorine, an ice-creamlike product in which vegetable oil replaces the milk fat. (If mellorine or filled milk is available in your state, make sure that the products are not made with coconut or palm oil—the two saturated vegetable fats.) Ironically, a few states that allow mellorine do not permit low-fat mellorine—a better choice because it contains less of all fats.

The Dairy Lobby

Some states also will not permit alternatives to cheese made with saturated milk fat; in 1978, when the Kraft Company began marketing a new line of cheese in which corn oil replaces much of the milk fat, it found the product illegal in eight states. North Dakota, South Dakota, Oregon, Michigan, Minnesota, Nebraska, Vermont, and Washington would not permit a cheese that doesn't help raise blood cholesterol levels.

Though federal regulations for minimum fat in dairy products are more enlightened than some state laws, federal policy on one food—margarine—also reflects the failure of policy to keep pace with scientific knowledge. Until 1950, federal law taxed any margarine colored yellow; consumers had to pay a premium for yellow margarine or settle for uncolored margarine that could be colored at home by hand. The growing power of soybean, corn, and cotton farmers helped repeal the tax three decades ago. But the repeal was not won without a major concession to butter: a new law making margarine an unlikely commodity in restaurants. The law requires restaurants serving margarine to post a notice on a wall or on the menu disclosing that margarine is served, and also to serve the margarine clearly marked or cut into triangles. No other food served in restaurants is subject to a double notification requirement. According to the National Restaurant Association, the dual requirement is just too much red tape—enough to encourage restaurants to simply serve butter. Because Americans eat about one-third of their meals away from home, this law props up the butter market considerably. Even a restaurant that serves margarine only on request must observe the double notification requirements. In some states—Wisconsin, for example—margarine may be served only if the patron requests it. Wisconsin law also prohibits the serving of margarine in state schools, hospitals, or prisons, unless ordered by a physician.

Federal agencies, the American Heart Association, restaurant and hotel trade groups, and, of course, vegetable oil interests, have favored changing the law to require only one form of notification on margarine, but the change has yet to pass Congress. The dairy lobby, alias National Milk Producers

Federation, has said it will agree to a change in the margarine restrictions only if laws about serving other dairy substitutes are adopted. The federation wants serving of items such as cream substitutes regulated if laws making use of margarine more likely are passed. Of all barriers to more progressive dairy policies, the federation's constituency—the dairy farmers—is by far the most powerful.

Dairy farmers number about 400,000 in the United States and in 1978 accounted for about $13 billion of the $111 billion in farm receipts. Obviously, this is a large industry, though cattle ranchers and cattle feeders outnumber the dairy farmers by almost a million. Yet, the dairy farmers often have more political clout, and experience and political geography account for their power. The dairy farmers, though fewer in number, are scattered throughout the country, while cattle ranchers are concentrated in a few regions. Congressmen from almost every state hear from dairy farmers, giving the industry a loud voice. Dairy farmers also organized for government assistance. before the cattle ranchers did; the dairymen first organized for government price supports in the 1930s, whereas cattle raising did not become an organized industry until after World War II. As a result, the dairy farmers are old hands at dealing with Congress, and all politicians know it. "The dairymen are organized and they're militant," John Connally warned Richard Nixon in one of the famous Watergate tapes.

The dairy industry is also known for its generosity with campaign contributions. Common Cause, a citizens' lobby, studied congressional financial records and reported that in 1976, dairy interests ranked second only to the American Medical Association in donations to congressional campaigns. More than a million dollars was donated to members of Congress—including $82,686 donated to eight of eleven members of the House agriculture subcommittee concerned with dairy legislation.

Not surprisingly, the dairy industry has sought to use its political influence to keep the lid on the heart disease findings. The publication of *Healthy People* (the Surgeon General's report), the *Dietary Goals* report, the USDA-HHS dietary guidelines, and the National Cancer Institute's recommendation to eat less fat show that this strategy has not always worked, but in other cases the dairy industry's muscle has successfully overpowered the scientist's word. The dairy farmers have their lobby group, the National Milk Producers Federation, to oppose congressional action to inform the public about diet and heart disease; the National Dairy Council to keep the dairy industry's viewpoint in schools, newspaper food sections, and professional circles; and the American Dairy Association to advertise high-fat dairy products. All three of these major dairy organizations have tried to muzzle the lower-fat message. State and local dairy groups have also done their part in their communities, with the same mixed results.

In 1971, the Senate Select Committee on Nutrition and Human Needs scheduled its first hearings on diet and heart disease. The staff spent several months researching the issue and inviting witnesses, but at the last minute, the hearing was canceled without explanation. Soon afterward, an angry letter to the editor of *The Washington Post* held the dairy industry responsible for cancellation of the heart disease hearing. "Examination of this problem, the most important health problem facing the nation, was prevented by the pressure of dairy producers on captive politicians," thundered the letter writer. He was Dr. Jean Mayer, the country's most famous nutritionist.

The dairy industry pleaded innocent to the charge. "I don't think we ever would have tried to interfere with the hearing schedule set up by the Congress," responded Pat Healy, secretary of the National Milk Producers Federation. But a source familiar with the events on Capitol Hill said that the federation had worked behind the scenes to postpone the hearing. According to that source, the group had objected because witnesses supporting the relation between saturated fat, cholesterol, and heart disease were scheduled for the first day of the hearings, while skeptics were not to appear until the second day. The National Milk Producers Federation did not want the believers granted a full day to speak unchallenged, and through one of its most loyal senators, Gaylord Nelson of Wisconsin, pressured to have the hearing postponed until a different scheduling system could be arranged. The federation cleverly pointed out that McGovern, who was seeking the 1972 presidential nomination, should not allow a hearing that would upset Wisconsin dairy farmers with the Wisconsin primary only a few months away. The hearings were postponed, and eventually rescheduled, sandwiching believers and nonbelievers back to back. But this hearing too was canceled, as it conflicted with the 1972 presidential campaign. Six years passed before the hearings on diet and heart disease finally took place.

The successful cancellation of the 1971 heart disease hearing might have been some consolation to the many Wisconsin dairy farmers, but not much. They already had plenty to be upset about. The possibility of a two-day Senate hearing on diet and heart disease was a small threat compared to the on-going efforts of the American Heart Association (AHA). Since 1961, the AHA national office and its many chapters throughout the country had been advocating a diet lower in saturated fat and cholesterol for the general public.

The dairy farmers wanted to silence the AHA. Around 1970, a group of Wisconsin dairy cooperatives threatened the national organization and its Wisconsin chapter with a multimillion-dollar lawsuit, alleging "misleading" advice. The dairy interests tried to convince the Wisconsin Heart Association that it could not raise money in a dairy state like Wisconsin if it supported the diet recommendations of the national office. (State chapters of the AHA depend on local contributions for much of their support.) The arm-twisting efforts were fairly successful.

Soon after the dairy cooperatives threatened legal action, the Wisconsin Heart Association formed a Task Force on Nutrition and Cardiovascular Disease in hopes of reaching a compromise. The executive director of the Dairy Council of Wisconsin, the state's chapter of the National Dairy Council, served on the task force. The task force heard testimony from all sides—including a presentation by the National Dairy Council headquarters—and ten months later, adopted a position on saturated fat, cholesterol, and heart disease that represented a conservative departure from the position of the American Heart Association's national office. This task force position paper became the official policy of the Wisconsin Heart Association, even though it contradicted the position of the national organization. The national organization had adopted a policy statement in 1965 advising the public to eat less saturated fat and cholesterol and "to apply these dietary recommendations early in life." The last recommendation in the 1965 national statement urged the public "to make sound food habits a 'family affair,' so that benefits of proper nutritional practices—including the avoidance of high blood fat levels—may accrue to all members of the family." Prevention of high blood cholesterol was the goal of the national office.

By comparison, the new position adopted by the Wisconsin Heart Association recommended changes in diet only after high blood cholesterol had developed—as if no harm were done until then. In a statement for the press, the Wisconsin Heart Association said: "If hypercholesterolemia [high blood cholesterol] is not identified as a risk factor in an individual, however, Wisconsin Heart does not recommend a low-cholesterol, low-fat diet to prevent heart attacks and strokes." The dairy industry was pleased. The Dairy Council of Wisconsin passed a formal resolution commending the Wisconsin chapter for its "wisdom" in recognizing that "diets to lower blood cholesterol . . . are not warranted for the general public." The Dairy Council's national office in Chicago also sent a letter of congratulations. Dairy cooperatives also passed resolutions commending the Wisconsin Heart Association for its new position. Most important of all, dairy interests dropped their threatened lawsuit.

The national headquarters of the American Heart Association, though, was appalled by the goings-on in Wisconsin and challenged the scientific basis for the watered-down position that its Wisconsin chapter had adopted. But science aside, the national office told the Wisconsin chapter that it could not adopt positions that contradicted those passed by the national board of directors. The warning fell on deaf ears. Convinced that reneging on its compromise with the dairy industry would bring lawsuits and impossible fund-raising conditions, the Wisconsin Heart Association has continued to abide by its separate and weaker position. The Wisconsin Heart Association also does not promote the link between diet and heart disease in its public relations efforts. Diet information is distributed only on request, and the toned-down policy statement and the Dairy Council resolution commending it are attached to every reply for diet advice. "We don't aggressively promote it [the diet-heart link] any more than [a Heart Association chapter in] a tobacco state would promote the tobacco message," acknowledged a high official of the Wisconsin Heart Association.

Wisconsin provides the most dramatic example of dairy efforts to silence criticism of milk fat, but the dairy industry has used its resources to promote fat in every state. Dairy farmers fund a national promotion organization, the American Dairy Association, to the tune of $3.5 million per year. Commercials sponsored by the American Dairy Association seem curiously oriented toward butter and milk, which is never described as skim or low-fat. Jane Holmes, the organization's advertising director, denied that the group deliberately advertises only high-fat dairy products, but acknowledged that her organization would not advertise skim milk as having half the calories of whole milk. "That is for the dairy processors, who can make more money by skimming [milk] and selling the cream, [to do] . . . We are representing farmers, their maximum interests," she said. With milk priced on its fat content, the American Dairy Association is probably correct that the farmers' interests are best served by selling the fat as well as the nonfat part of the milk.

Though the American Dairy Association says it has no official policy against advertising low-fat dairy products, a California professional group has had such a policy since 1971. The California Milk Producers Advisory Board, a state-assisted promotional arm of California dairymen, was sponsoring TV commercials, and the original plans featured celebrities promoting milk products—including skim and low-fat varieties. The group's advertising committee later decided to keep words like *skim* and *low-fat* off the airwaves. According to minutes of a 1971 meeting, it happened like this:

Following a break for lunch, the Committee drove to KGO-TV station, where they reviewed the Pat Boone, Vikki Carr, and Dear Abby commercials. The use of low-fat, skim, and non-fat milk terms in the commercials was discussed thoroughly from both a producer-Advisory Board relationship and a consumer marketing viewpoint. Fred Manley described what could be done to edit the commercials and the limitations concerning changing statements made by the celebrities.

Santos moved, seconded by Thompson, that we establish a policy that new commercials do not contain any reference to non-fat, skim, or low-fat milks and that emphasis be placed upon whole milk, except for the Pat Boone radio and television commercials. The Boone TV commercial is to be edited to definitely remove the "weight control" section and the non-fat and skim words, if possible. Following discussion, the motion passed.

The dairy representatives are aware, though, that advertising alone will not keep demand for milk fat where they want it. It helps if the public believes that high-fat dairy products are nutritious, and this is the purpose of the National Dairy Council and its 128 local chapters. As *Dairyman,* a trade magazine, editorialized, "It's important to understand the unique role the Dairy Council plays in promoting milk. The Dairy Council does no paid consumer advertising. That noncommercial status is important. As a highly respected nutrition education entity its programs give the dairy industry entry into areas difficult to penetrate with straight product promotion, especially the schools and medical-dental professions. . . ."

Headquartered in suburban Chicago, the national office of the Dairy Council thrives on a $2-million budget contributed mostly by dairy farmers. Milk processors also contribute a small portion of its budget. The Dairy Council's materials are promoted to the nation's schools by local chapters in 128 U.S. cities; these local affiliates, also funded by milk interests, add another $12 million to the budget for spreading the Dairy Council message. A few paragraphs in *Milk Still Makes the Difference,* the Dairy Council's self-profile, epitomize its position on saturated fat and cholesterol:

> Members of the dairy industry are as susceptible to coronary heart disease as anyone else. Certainly we would all like to see the defeat of this killer in our society. But we hate to hear our food products indicted unjustly. . . .
>
> Therefore, research supported through NDC's grant-in-aid program seeks to set the record straight about the influence of diet on heart disease. We cannot rest until our product is completely vindicated and put into proper perspective.

The Dairy Council's materials on nutrition live up to this credo. Whole milk, ice cream, hard cheese, and butter dominate its publications, which revolve around the Basic Four and nutrient requirements. Pictures of skim milk, ice milk, or yogurt and cottage cheese cartons labeled "low-fat" are rare, if not nonexistent in its materials. A few examples show the same high-fat advice preached to young and old:

• *Food: Your Choice,* Level One, the Dairy Council's curriculum package for elementary schools, is a large box filled with colorful materials, among them posters about making milk shakes and pancakes. The recipes call for ice cream, butter, yogurt, and milk not labeled low-fat. The kit also includes mimeograph masters for making handouts. Of the numerous handouts, none feature low-fat dairy foods. Only cream cheese, milk, ice cream, and butter are pictured.

206

• Teachers also receive special guides to supplement the students' materials. The teacher's guide *Ice Cream for You and Me* advises: "Ice cream is a healthful food that is made from milk and cream along with other good foods." Another teacher's guide exemplifies the Dairy Council's devotion to milk fat with this advice: "Drink milk at every meal and have some in foods like these: cheese, ice cream, baked custard, bowl of cream of tomato soup, with a pat of butter melting on top." Cottage cheese, ice milk, low-fat yogurt go unmentioned.

• Teenagers can choose from the Dairy Council's *A Boy and His Physique* or *A Girl and Her Figure*. The workbook *A Girl and Her Figure and You* lists milk as the first snack suggestion, but with a qualification—it should be whole milk. "[Drink] whole milk most of the time, skim milk part of the time if you need to lose weight," reads the booklet. In addition to allowing skim milk only "part of the time" and only for overweight girls, the Dairy Council plugs "a medium dip of ice cream with berries, chopped cranberries, or other fruit, unsweetened" as "Stay-slim sundaes." Also listed in the lower-calorie section are balls of cream cheese softened with cream or fruit juice, rolled in chopped peanuts and served in fruit.

The Dairy Council has even been known to insist on whole milk for dieters. *The Basic Four Way to Safe and Sensible Weight Control,* published by a Pennsylvania chapter, prescribes a glass of whole milk and a pat of butter at every meal on its reducing plan. And if this reducing plan isn't a blatant enough plug for unnecessary milk fat, the leaflet lists whole milk as the first entry on a list of low-calorie foods. Skim milk—with half as many calories as whole milk—isn't listed. And topping the list of "lower-caloried" snacks is—(what else?)—ice cream. Ice milk, with less fat than ice cream and fewer calories, has been relegated to the same status as skim milk—completely forgotten.

Centering on the Basic Four and the Recommended Dietary Allowances for protein, vitamins, and minerals, Dairy Council publications almost never mention the heart scientist's advice to think about saturated fat and cholesterol as well as nutrients. The few exceptions are some publications designed to make you wonder if the American Heart Association knows what it's talking about.

One of the Dairy Council's tactics to diffuse concern about milk fat is acknowledging only its cholesterol but not its saturated fat. This strategy—also used well by the meat and chocolate industries—can fool people who associate only cholesterol in food with cholesterol in the blood, unaware that saturated fat is the prime influence on blood cholesterol levels. The *Pocket Guide to CHOLESTEROL Counting,* a publication of the Southampton, Pennsylvania, Dairy Council, lists only the cholesterol content of foods and labels the entire group of dairy products, including heavy cream, butter, ice cream, and sour cream, as *"High* in nutrient value and 'best-quality' protein. Modest in number of calories!" Because milk fat contains only moderate amounts of cholesterol, foods like cheese and ice cream, which are rich in saturated fat, look blissfully innocuous. Needless to say, Dairy Councils do not publish a *Pocket Guide to SATURATED FAT Counting.*

The national office of the Dairy Council also uses this approach. Its pamphlet, *Coronary Heart Disease: Risk Factors and the Diet Debate,* devotes a full page to the cholesterol content of foods, but saturated fat content is nowhere to be found. The Dairy Council apparently hoped that this technique would maintain the image of high-fat dairy products. An internal memo describing the booklet says: "Charts show the amounts of cholesterol in average cooked servings of animal meat, fish, seafood, poultry and eggs, desserts and dairy foods. Dairy products are seen to be lower in cholesterol content than other animal foods and many desserts." And while the Dairy Council's promotional letter touts the booklet's "objective information," the internal memo acknowledges that the booklet was prepared in part "to provide the dairy industry with a means to answer criticism aimed at dairy foods, specifically milk fat, in relation to heart disease." The pamphlet does admit that "many" medical researchers favor a diet with no more than 10 percent of its calories from saturated fat, but because it gives no information on how to achieve such a diet (and recommends the usual Basic Four), the typical American diet sounds like the prescription for preventing heart disease.

The Dairy Council produces not just curriculum materials, but also a nutrition column for newspapers, public service announcements for TV and radio, and two annual conferences for food editors. For the most part, the Dairy Council has eluded criticism of its outdated approach to nutrition and its distorted presentation of facts about diet and heart disease. In fact, the Dairy Council remains the major supplier of nutrition information materials for schools. Its staff in 128 cities often provide workshops to train teachers in the Dairy Council's brand of nutrition. Even federal funds earmarked for nutrition education are spent on the Dairy Council's wares. Since 1977, Congress has allocated $15 to $27 million per year for the Nutrition Education Training Program— a program intended to educate teachers, children, and school food service personnel about good nutrition. Each state receives 25 to 50 cents per child for nutrition education.

Unfortunately, most states have considered the Dairy Council a fine source of nutrition information. Of the forty-two states that submitted their 1978 program plans to the USDA, thirty-nine indicated that Dairy Council materials had been in use before the Nutrition Education and Training Program began, and twenty-nine implied that the federal funds would be used to continue purchase of Dairy Council materials. Ironically, nutrition education specialists in Iowa, Delaware, and Idaho expressed concern about the fat content of the children's diets, only to praise the Dairy Council materials as a welcome part of their educational program.

Why has the Dairy Council succeeded despite its outdated and self-serving approach to nutrition? One reason is that few groups have tried to compete with the Dairy Council; its prices are hard to beat thanks to dairy industry subsidies. The Dairy Council also promotes its materials exceptionally well. But low prices, lack of competition, and good salesmanship aren't the only reasons that the Dairy Council has remained number one in the nutrition education world. The group's success is due largely to its former track record.

During its first five decades, the Dairy Council's message was accepted wisdom in scientific circles. In those days, the Dairy Council did not have to choose between two masters; scientists' beliefs of the time enabled the group to serve both the public and the dairy farmers by advocating the Basic Four. Only as a consensus about diet and heart disease developed during the past twenty years was the Dairy Council forced to choose between two masters, and not surprisingly, it has sided with the hand that feeds it. Unfortunately for the public, the Dairy Council is still riding on the esteem accorded to it in earlier days, and this once-deserved respect has allowed it to keep face among educators and journalists who are not always aware of changing attitudes in science.

The story of the National Dairy Council epitomizes the history of dairy policy in this country. During the first half of the twentieth century, policymakers and farm groups lived at a time when science considered the dairy farmer's interest and public health interests one and the same. Serving two masters was simple then, for both were served by the same policies. But as nutrition science matured, a much more difficult situation—where farm interests are sometimes at odds with health interests—has evolved.

Still the dairy farmers remain in a good position. State and national laws protect the milk fat market. Government agencies and private groups have not provided nutrition education materials on the massive scale needed to counter those distributed by the Dairy Council. Most important, the government guarantees farmers a buyer for every drop of milk fat they produce. Unless government dairy policies change, dairy farmers will have no incentive to reduce their production of surplus fat, or to promote low-fat dairy products. And one master—the dairy industry—will be served at the expense of the other—the public.

11

The Egg Lobby

Replacing old ideas with new ones is an endless process in science. Today, the science of nutrition is engaged in a tug-of-war between scholars who recommend any vitamin-rich food and a newer generation that thinks not just about a food's nutrient value, but about its fat and cholesterol, too. But ironically, the current old school was once a new school fighting to be heard. When some scientists first proposed that food contained tiny amounts of the nutrients now known as vitamins, the scientific mainstream laughed heartily in disbelief.

Between 1840 and 1910, scientists generally accepted that protein, fats, carbohydrates, and certain minerals were the only nutrients necessary for health. All forms of fat were considered the same—the official word was that 50 grams of lard was no different from 50 grams of butter. But during the last forty years of this period—from 1871 to 1910, a few scientists proposed that food contained more than the four recognized classes of nutrients. They had experimental evidence to support their conclusions. But some of nutrition's most prominent scholars resisted, unwilling to accept the possibility that additional nutrients existed in food.

The innovators of the time were people such as Elmer

McCollum and Marguerite Davis, the first to publish a paper about the elusive substance in milk fat and egg yolk that was essential to the proper growth of rats. It was the first demonstration that all fats were not alike in nutritive value. Some fats had something essential that other fats lacked. That something, of course, proved to be vitamin A.

While McCollum and Davis continued to study vitamins, McCollum's former teacher, Dr. Lafayette Mendel, and his Yale colleague, Dr. Thomas Osborne, became leaders in protein research. Osborne and Mendel were among the first to show that, like fats, all proteins were not the same. Using a technique that later became a classic method, these two researchers found that the young rats fed milk proteins as the only protein in their diets grew properly and well, while rats fed only one of the proteins in corn or wheat failed to thrive. Later research showed that egg protein also produced excellent growth in rats. Scientists determined that differences in the amino acid content of foods accounted for the results. Proteins are giant complexes of the smaller units called amino acids, and animal proteins contain higher concentrations of the eight amino acids needed by man than do vegetable proteins.

When Osborne and Mendel first published their results in 1914, they were not on good terms with Elmer McCollum. There had been a controversy the year before over who had first discovered vitamin A. Only a few months after McCollum and Davis published their first paper on vitamin A, Osborne and Mendel published similar findings and attacked the McCollum and Davis work as unconvincing. Personal hostilities remained for many years as a result of this rift over who had produced the first solid evidence of an essential growth factor in milk fat and egg yolk. After publication of the two competing papers, wrote McCollum in his autobiography, "There was always a coolness in the manner of Osborne and Mendel toward me. It caused me great regret."

But though Osborne and Mendel did not have friendly relations with McCollum, their work could not have complemented his more beautifully. It was McCollum who had dubbed whole milk and egg yolk "protective foods" in honor of their vitamin A content. The spectacular differences in growth among young rats fed only milk or egg proteins versus rats fed grain proteins gave even more currency to the "protective foods" label. By 1920, nutritionists were sold on milk and eggs for two reasons: for their vitamin A content and for their impressive protein value. The 1932 discovery of kwashiorkor, a devastating disease marked by protein deficiency, further persuaded nutritionists of the importance of milk and eggs in the diet.

Spurred by the incidence of kwashiorkor among children in developing countries, scientists began to study not just protein needs of rats, but those of humans as well. Research found differences between growing rats and man, but one striking similarity stood out. For both, protein needs can be met more easily with eggs or milk than with only grains. Meeting protein needs of young children with only vegetable proteins requires know-how, a risk most nutritionists feel is not worth taking. Children need more protein per pound of body weight than adults, and for this reason, they are particularly vulnerable to protein deficiency disease.

In 1938, researchers at the University of Rochester found that of the two most-studied animal proteins, egg had a slight edge over milk when these foods provided the only protein in the diet. Their findings were upheld in 1965, when a joint committee of the United Nations Food and Agriculture Organization and the World Health Organization reviewed research on human protein needs and concluded that the proteins of egg and human milk most closely matched the pattern of amino acids required by man. Egg protein became the standard against which other proteins were measured.

The selection of eggs as the standard for judging protein was probably the most favorable conclusion ever reached about eggs. Eggs had reached their pinnacle in the nutritionists' esteem. But trouble was just around the corner.

The trouble was that the egg, so rich in protein and vitamins, was also rich in cholesterol. During the 1950s, scientists had been unimpressed with the effect of food cholesterol on blood cholesterol levels. Studies had shown no effect of large doses of pure cholesterol crystals on blood cholesterol levels. Almost by accident, a team of scientists later learned that the body would absorb the cholesterol crystals used in laboratory studies only if accompanied by fat. Pure cholesterol given with fat caused definite increases in blood cholesterol levels, prompting scientists to reconsider their earlier conclusions. To be sure that the cholesterol crystals weren't giving misleading results, they studied common cholesterol-containing foods—including the much-touted egg.

In 1961, William Connor and his colleagues at the University of Iowa published an experiment showing a notable effect of cholesterol-rich egg yolk on blood cholesterol levels. In 1965, the same year that protein experts from the United Nations and World Health Organization adopted egg as the protein standard, scientific journals published two classic papers again demonstrating a cholesterol-raising effect of egg yolk. Three University of Minnesota researchers—Drs. Ancel Keys, Joseph Anderson, and Francisco Grande—reported that a diet with 380 mg of egg yolk cholesterol per day caused an average blood cholesterol level 16 mg higher than a diet with only 50 mg cholesterol. Dr. Mark Hegsted and his colleagues at the Harvard School of Public Health found that each 100 mg of egg yolk cholesterol raised blood cholesterol levels of adult men an average of 4 to 5 mg. As a result of these studies and still others, the American Heart Association amended its diet advice to include not just reduction of saturated fat, but of food cholesterol also.

But scientists who had been enamored of eggs for more than fifty years reacted angrily to the Heart Association's advice to kick the two-egg-a-day habit. (The Heart Association recommends about three yolks per week, particularly for men.) An assortment of arguments to preserve the unblemished reputation of eggs poured out. Those unwilling to change their views would point out that cholesterol is needed for development of the brain and nervous system. "Will the American Heart Association defend the potential malpractice suits brought against it if and when a generation of low-IQ students develop from its unproven dietary recommendations?" demanded Dr. Kurt Oster, a Connecticut physician.

Opponents of the American Heart Association lauded cholesterol not just for its benefit to the brain and nerves, but to all cells of the body. "Cholesterol is an absolute essential for our bodies all through life," wrote Dr. Roger Williams, a University of Texas professor who discovered one of the B vitamins, pantothenic acid. Dr. Helen Guthrie, a nutritionist at Pennsylvania State University, concurred. "Since a certain amount of cholesterol is essential for the synthesis of sex hormones, for the transport of essential fatty acids, and as a constituent of the skin and covering nerve fibers, it must be considered a normal body constituent," she wrote in her textbook, *Introductory Nutrition*.

At face value, the arguments were true. Cholesterol *is* essential for body cells—particularly for the brain and nervous system. It *is* needed for synthesis of sex hormones. But the arguments made a subtle implication that is not true: that the cholesterol in foods is innocent of the charges against it because the body requires cholesterol. Scientists have never found that the body needs cholesterol from food. "As far as we can determine, all of us would do just as well if we had no cholesterol in the diet," National Heart, Lung, and Blood Institute director Robert Levy explained to puzzled senators at a hearing. "Cholesterol can be made by all of the cells in the body so we don't need to take in any." And, the cholesterol in food can be more than unnecessary—too much of it can help put blood cholesterol levels in the danger zone.

But the old school insisted that eating fewer eggs would bring dire consequences—as Kurt Oster predicted "a generation of low-IQ students." Vitamin discoverer Roger Williams warned, "Most of our good foods contain substantial amounts of cholesterol, and if we try to eliminate cholesterol consumption we sacrifice good nutrition. . . . Anyone who deliberately avoids cholesterol in his

215

diet may be inadvertently courting heart disease." And when not predicting doom from lower-cholesterol diets, some scientists simply denied that the cholesterol in eggs raises blood cholesterol levels. They'd quote the old studies in which cholesterol crystals were fed without fat as proof that food cholesterol doesn't count. They'd cite survey studies in which scientists could not show a correlation between blood cholesterol and the amount of cholesterol that people reported eating. They'd argue that the body simply compensates for cholesterol eaten by making less of its own.

But using these arguments to absolve food cholesterol meant ignoring other kinds of evidence. It meant ignoring the retractions of the cholesterol crystals studies written by the very people who did the experiments. It meant ignoring extensive scientific commentaries showing that within the U.S. population, diets do not differ enough from person to person to show a relationship between blood cholesterol levels and food habits reported on questionnaires. It meant ignoring sophisticated experiments showing that while the body does decrease its own cholesterol production when cholesterol is added to the diet, the balancing mechanism usually does not compensate for all of the cholesterol eaten. Some of it often lands in the blood, as closely monitored experiments showed. But the opponents of the American Heart Association ignored these studies too. They also ignored a 1974 National Academy of Sciences review advising that eggs no longer be used as the protein standard. New research indicates that egg protein is not as ideal as once thought, though it is still high-quality.

It wasn't just anybody who was carefully selecting arguments to challenge the American Heart Association's position. The arguments were presented by some of the leaders in the nutrition field, and so the nation listened. And no one was listening quite as closely as the egg producers.

Egg producers were shocked by the American Heart Association's statement favoring fewer eggs in the diet, just as meat and dairy interests were dumbfounded by its recommendations to restrict meat and dairy fats. But the egg producers were especially sensitive about the Heart Association's advice. Egg consumption had been falling slowly in the United States since 1950, and the 1965 warnings about their cholesterol content looked like more fuel for a roller coaster that was already headed downhill. (Beef consumption, by contrast, had been rising steadily.) The egg industry, as a breakfast industry, was suffering from changing life-styles that had made a sit-down breakfast a thing of the past. The new American life-style had not victimized the traditional meat-and-potatoes dinner in the same way that it had upstaged the egg.

The American Heart Association had added insult to injury, and the egg industry was frantic. As the years went by and other expert committees added their voices to the Heart Association's, the egg industry became more frantic still. Egg consumption continued to fall. In the early 1970s, a group of alarmed egg producers formed an organization to do combat with the Heart Association and its allies. They called themselves the National Commission on Egg Nutrition (NCEN).

The NCEN was worried and angry, and its officials, accustomed to only glowing comments about eggs, were greenhorns at fighting criticism. They groped for solutions, and finally, chose advertising.

Instead of trying the soft sell—just touting the good points in eggs—NCEN opted for the hard sell. NCEN ads in *The Wall Street Journal* and other daily newspapers attacked the diet-heart advice head-on. "There is absolutely no scientific evidence that eating eggs, even in quantity, will increase the risk of a heart attack" declared a typical ad. The ad campaign also featured six "facts" about cholesterol:

1. Cholesterol is the building block of sex hormones.
2. Cholesterol is needed for the nerves to transmit their impulses throughout the body.

3. Cholesterol is essential for life for every cell in the body.
4. The less cholesterol one eats, the more cholesterol the body produces because a person's system needs cholesterol.
5. The normal person's body will eliminate just about the same amount of cholesterol as that eaten.
6. Eggs contain cholesterol—as do all foods of animal origin—*and are the richest source of protein in human nutrition.* [Emphasis from original]

The ads offered a free booklet about cholesterol that elaborated on the six arguments. NCEN thought it was on the right track in its efforts to sway public opinion.

But the next thing the NCEN officials knew, they were in trouble—expensive trouble. The American Heart Association had complained to the Federal Trade Commission that the NCEN ads were false and deceptive, and the FTC listened. An investigation began, one which led to a formal complaint against the NCEN and its advertising agency, Richard Weiner, Inc. Five of the nation's most respected heart disease researchers agreed to testify before the FTC that the NCEN ads were misleading.

The NCEN was up to its knees in legal trouble, and its attorney admitted from the start that the chances of beating the lawsuit on scientific grounds were almost nil. The NCEN officials could not understand why. The ads, after all, were not their own words. The NCEN's defense of eggs was little more than an ad agency's version of the subtle arguments used by change-resistant nutritionists. It was the widely used textbook *Introductory Nutrition* that used the first of NCEN's arguments—that cholesterol "must be considered a normal body constituent" because it is needed for synthesis of sex hormones. Roger Williams, the noted vitamin pioneer, had supplied argument number three—that cholesterol is essential to life—in his book *Nutrition Against Disease.* The textbook *Nutrition in Nursing,* also written by respected nutritionists, offered a version of arguments four and five, which assured that the normal person's body compensated for food cholesterol consumed. The NCEN could make no claims of originality for its arguments. The arguments had come from the mouth of nutrition's old school.

Laws do not regulate the arguments of textbook writers. But the same arguments used in advertising, for the purposes of defending financial interests, present another story. It was a story that involved the NCEN in a long and costly legal battle to defend itself against a serious government lawsuit.

NCEN's lawyer had correctly predicted that a scientific defense would not stand up in court. As the case progressed, NCEN's scientific arguments took a beating. But the NCEN's efforts at a First Amendment defense also failed; the FTC ruled that the NCEN ads were not protected by the Constitutional guarantee of freedom of speech. In the final ruling, the FTC prohibited the NCEN from running ads that deny the link between cholesterol and heart disease, as well as any ads that represent cholesterol as essential to health. The FTC also ordered corrective advertisements and ruled that the NCEN must disclose its industry sponsorship in every ad. The name "National Commission on Egg Nutrition," charged the FTC, "implies an impartial, independent, quasi-governmental health commission, when in fact it is an association of persons engaged in the egg industry."

The NCEN appealed the FTC's ruling, but lost. On appeal, though, the requirement for corrective advertising was dropped. The group tried to have the Supreme Court hear the case, but to no avail. It had exhausted its legal resources, much emotional energy, and much of its treasury on a losing battle. NCEN officials were bitter, but determined to carry on their war with the American Heart Association. But it was clear that a new approach, and really, a new organization, was needed.

The egg industry took its war to Congress, seeking a platform for defending eggs that would be better-funded than the NCEN had been. Egg industry strategists wanted to harness as much of the industry's strength as possible, and to do so, proposed that Congress help create a national egg promotion organization.

219

Funds for the organization would come from taxes on egg producers, and the USDA would be charged with administering the plan.

The egg industry's representatives knew that if anyone were to oppose their plan, it would be the American Heart Association or professional societies of heart researchers. But the advocates of the egg promotions bill sidestepped that problem with money for research. Promoters of the Egg Research and Promotion Act pledged that part of the funds collected would be made available for university research. There was no better way to stop scientific opposition in its tracks. Research money is the magic word in science, and by promising to provide it, the egg industry all but had the heart researchers lobbying for the bill.

It was not the first time that the egg industry had funded research. Before the American Egg Board was born, other egg industry groups had supported university research. The NCEN had funded research on the effect of eggs on blood cholesterol levels. California egg producers had supported similar research. The Wallace Genetic Foundation, a private group funded in part by egg magnate H. B. Wallace, had also supported heart disease research—much of it done at the Harlan Moore Research Foundation at the University of Illinois. The director of the Moore Foundation, Dr. Fred Kummerow, had testified on behalf of the NCEN at the FTC hearings. Some of these studies provided the industry with what it wanted: seemingly scientific research to challenge the American Heart Association's position. Unfortunately for the public, the studies were too often poor ones that would be less likely to show an effect of eggs on blood cholesterol than well-designed studies.

Two of the egg industry's experiments were done at the University of Missouri, and at face value they appear to show that eggs have no significant effect on blood cholesterol. Dr. Margaret Flynn and her colleagues asked a group of men to add or omit eggs from their usual diets, and the researchers reported no significant effects on blood cholesterol occurred, despite the requested changes in the diet. "Serious design flaws prevent interpretation of the results," wrote the National Heart, Lung, and Blood Institute in a critique of these experiments and others that the egg industry claims supports its case. "The diet instructions were so vague and the control and assessment of diet so poor that it is entirely possible that over all or most of each twelve-week period, any effects of changes in the dietary cholesterol may have been obliterated by the fact that there may have been little or no difference in dietary cholesterol intakes and/or differences in dietary fats."

The National Heart, Lung, and Blood Institute also criticized a study by Dr. Grant Slater and his colleagues at the University of California at Los Angeles. California egg producers had funded this study, which the NHLBI said "suffered numerous serious faults which would be expected to prevent observation of an effect." The NHLBI also interpreted the results differently than the researchers, who said that eggs had not affected their subjects' blood cholesterol levels. "Despite the author's conclusions and all the serious flaws in the study, the results do indicate an effect of egg cholesterol on plasma [blood] cholesterol," said the NHLBI. Likewise, the NHLBI did not give a clean bill of health to some research from the University of Illinois, the biggest recipient of egg industry research money. "The results from Urbana, which showed no response of plasma cholesterol to additional dietary cholesterol, were meaningless and should be discarded," said the critique, criticizing the five-hour duration of the experiment as ridiculously short.

Egg industry representatives apparently did not care about the quality of the research—they tried to get as much mileage as possible from the seemingly favorable results. The California Egg Program, supporter of the University of California egg study, assigned its advertising agency to publicize the results of the study. The agency did its job well, generating "eggs don't raise cholesterol" publicity through radio and TV interviews, press conferences, and a clever plan of inserting flyers describing the study's results into four to five million egg cartons in the Los Angeles area.

Not surprisingly, egg interests repeatedly mentioned the three studies in their efforts to refute the *Dietary Goals for the United States* proposed by the Senate Select Committee on Nutrition and Human Needs. (It was Senator McGovern, chairman of the committee, who asked the NHLBI to comment on the validity of the studies.) Various egg industry representatives sent copies of the studies to Senate staff to refute the recommendations on reducing cholesterol in the diet.

Egg producers waged quite a campaign against the *Dietary Goals*. Sometimes it was hardball politics: the Indiana State Poultry Association, for instance, wrote to Congressman Adam Benjamin requesting his "assistance and cooperation in stopping immediately the distribution of the highly controversial report." In addition to seeking withdrawal of the report, the egg industry generated scores of letters requesting a public forum for its arguments. The senators soon agreed that the egg producers, like the meat industry, could have a hearing to rebut the report.

At the hearing in July 1977, the egg industry did not succeed very well at changing the senators' minds about the scientific accuracy of the report. Jack Dubose, a representative of the United Egg Producers, ran through the studies that supposedly absolved eggs. The committee was not convinced; the second edition of the *Dietary Goals* recommended the same 300 mg limitation on cholesterol as the first edition. However, the second edition did point out that, in general, men have to be stricter about their egg consumption than children or premenopausal women. Still, the revised report added that "in suggesting that the cholesterol [guideline] might be eased for young children, premenopausal women, and the elderly in order to obtain the nutritional benefits of additional eggs, the Select Committee does remain concerned as to what happens when the period of reduced risk is over and possible cumulative effects from the diet take place." The egg industry was not happy with the revised report.

There was consolation, though, that the industry's political clout had convinced a few of the senators to give only equivocal support to the second edition of the *Dietary Goals*. As described

222

earlier, Illinois Senator Charles Percy feared losing the farm vote in an upcoming election. He wrote a foreword to the new edition giving at best lukewarm support to the report. Senators Zorinsky of Nebraska and Schweiker of Pennsylvania co-signed his foreword, and Kansas Senator Dole wrote his own that likewise appeared at most a half-hearted endorsement.

In addition to fighting the *Dietary Goals,* the egg industry opposed the National Consumer Nutrition Information Act, a bill sponsored by Congressman Fred Richmond of New York. The bill would have allocated $10 million to expand government nutrition education programs. The United Egg Producers tried to give a scientific appearance to its arguments against the bill. "The current state of the scientific community is quite unsettled over the diet–cholesterol theory. There are reputable, independent, dedicated scientists on both sides of this controversy," wrote Betty Vorhies, a lobbyist for the group.

The Poultry and Egg Institute likewise opposed the bill for fear that the proposed nutrition education effort would include warnings against eating too much saturated fat and cholesterol. "Will information on such controversial subjects as the relationship of sugar, fat, cholesterol, alcohol, ruffage [sic] and salt to heart disease, cancer and other 'killer diseases' be used?" demanded Richard Ammon, vice-president of the organization. "The [Poultry and Egg] Institute is reluctant to support an educational measure until appropriate safeguards regarding the information content and the maintenance of freedom of dietary choice are established in the bill."

The egg industry had its way: the bill died in the House Agriculture Committee. Meat and egg lobbyists were credited with its defeat. Whether the egg industry had defeated the bill with its scientific arguments or with its power of money and votes was anybody's guess, but one thing was certain. In the process of trying to convince others that eggs have no relationship to blood cholesterol levels, egg industry representatives have deluded themselves and the farmers who they are entrusted to serve.

"I do believe that the myth of the contribution of the egg to coronary heart disease will be dispelled in my lifetime, and [that] my grandchildren will come to recognize me as a reasonably honest man," egg producer Norman Hecht told senators at the egg industry's hearing. After twenty years of research on diet and heart disease, the egg industry was still chasing its rainbow, fervently believing that one day the cholesterol warnings would vanish into thin air. The industry had constructed so many defenses that it insulated itself from any evidence contrary to its cause.

Throughout the years of heart disease research, leading scientists and physicians had tried to help the egg industry understand the effect of eggs on blood cholesterol. In 1971, the American Heart Association's medical director, Dr. Campbell Moses, met with egg industry representatives to explain his organization's position. In statements that followed the meeting, egg organizations claimed that Moses "could cite no valid scientific studies" linking eggs to heart disease. According to the egg industry, Moses said that the Heart Association's advice on eggs was based on "clinical opinion." Moses calls the claims "not at all" what was said. "They came with their minds made up and left thinking they had heard the same," said Moses.

Five years later, American Egg Board officials met with Dr. Robert Levy, director of the National Heart, Lung, and Blood Institute. At the meeting, Levy told the egg producers that research had established an effect of egg yolk on blood cholesterol. They refused to believe him. The American Egg Board's research consultant, former journalist Robert Fisher, wrote to Nebraska Senator Carl Curtis complaining about Levy's position:

Until last October, we believed that the National Heart, Lung, and Blood Institute had no part in perpetuating the cholesterol humbug. However, in conference with Dr. Robert Levy, chief of that organization, we heard him unequivocally state his support of AHA [American Heart Association] anti-egg pronouncements. Challenged to produce the research references to substantiate his statement, he did so. However, one would need to stretch the imagination considerably to believe they comprise an indictment of eggs.

About a year after meeting with Levy, one of the participants, H. B. Wallace, heard that an NHLBI experiment had shown no effect of eggs on blood cholesterol levels. Wallace, the developer of a hybrid chick widely used on egg farms, wrote to Levy, accusing him of suppressing vital research findings. In his letter, he tried to frighten Levy with predictions of retaliation from Congress if the study, conducted by Dr. Peter Herbert, were not quickly made public:

> Under present circumstances, there's just no way a show-down in the cholesterol matter can be avoided. The time to set the potential aside would have been last year, in the testimony before the [Senate] Select Committee [on Nutrition and Human Needs]. If McGovern had been told that the entire matter is up in the air, there'd be no problem at present. . . .
>
> You evidently knew of Herbert's findings weeks before you met with us, and you certainly knew of them when you testified before the Select Committee. We can forgive you, because it's the same reception we've received nearly everywhere, but do you believe McGovern will excuse your putting him out on a limb, with no graceful line of retreat? With the personal setbacks he's had, he's liable to be extremely harsh with anyone who misleads him.
>
> We don't know why you chose to black out information about Peter Herbert's findings . . . we don't know why you haven't credited knowledge dug up under your own super-vision. If you've been hesitating to issue the information because Herbert's findings haven't been published, you're risking your neck on a strictly scientific procedure which has no validity so far as the general public is concerned. To withhold critical information amounts to an indictable of-

fense in the eyes of individuals desperately seeking to improve their own health. Do you believe you can safely escape the consequences of your decision to withhold this information?

"The choice to seek publication of this research was and still is a decision of Dr. Herbert," responded Levy to Wallace's charges. "The fact that Dr. Herbert's data is not published is probably justified," continued Levy. "There are many problems in the study design. I believe Dr. Herbert recognized these short-comings. . . ." And contrary to Wallace's belief that the study had shown no effect of eggs on cholesterol levels, Levy's letter noted, "Even with the design faults there was an increase in plasma cholesterol when eggs were introduced and a fall when they were removed."

But the response from Levy, like other efforts to explain research to the egg industry, fell on deaf ears. Several months later, Wallace's close assistant, Robert Fisher, gave a sugar-coated but twisted version of the story to his audience at the annual meeting of the Pacific Egg and Poultry Association. "Tests in the National Heart, Blood, and Lung Institute [sic] have put the icing on the cake. NHLBI scientists found no effect on serum cho-lesterol from feeding as many as six eggs a day," Fisher told the thrilled crowd. "We hope the results will be published. The scientific world can question results secured with egg industry money. But it can't question results secured with everyone's money, with public funds."

Fisher went further still, assuring the egg producers that a high egg intake produces a "slow, inexorable improvement" in the level of HDL-cholesterol. Ironically, when one of the American Egg Board's research studies was published six months later, it showed that very high egg intakes changed the HDL in a way that might promote atherosclerosis. No matter what was said, the story from the egg industry was the same.

The industry not only refused to listen to what it didn't want to hear, but threatened legal action against those who talked too loudly. After reporting in his newspaper column that the American Heart Association had advised restriction of cholesterol intake, Dr. Lawrence Lamb heard from the egg industry lawyers. In one of his columns, Lamb told readers of the effort to silence him, revealing that a legal firm representing the egg industry had sent him a letter "apparently attempting to intimidate me." According to Lamb the letter alluded to legal action, and charged that his column was "most detrimental to the egg industry."

Lamb wasn't the only one to receive a threat. When the USDA published its pamphlet, *Nutrition and Your Health: Dietary Guidelines for Americans,* in 1980, the United Egg Producers requested that its distribution be halted because of the recommendation to avoid "too much cholesterol." "I ask on behalf of all egg producers that you cease distribution of this detrimental and inaccurate brochure and that future USDA nutrition publications reflect all data regarding the diet-heart controversy," Albert Pope, the group's executive vice-president, wrote to Agriculture Secretary Bob Bergland. "We respectfully urge and request that the *Dietary Guidelines* be immediately modified to represent a more accurate, and thus positive, portrayal of eggs. However, your failure to address our concerns, herein outlined, will necessarily result in our using every available resource to change the direction that the Department [of Agriculture] appears to be taking on nutrition issues." At their 1980 annual meeting, the United Egg Producers approved a program to combat the dietary guidelines. According to the trade journal *The Poultry Times,* legal, congressional, and scientific approaches were planned.

While the egg industry relied on defensive tactics to protect its interests, alternative approaches were left by the wayside. The industry might have sought solutions to the cholesterol content of egg yolk, but this road went unexplored. More than one individual had urged the industry to attempt a low-cholesterol egg, but no one said it more eloquently than Senator Richard Schweiker did at the egg industry's hearing to rebut the *Dietary Goals:*

[Other] industries have faced the same problem. How have they responded? Milk industry—my grandfather produced milk—is selling skim milk. They responded to their dilemma. So has the yogurt industry. Iced tea—it is called "iced tea light." You get 30 calories per drink compared to 60. They have marked down the sugar, reduced the problem and given an option.

Beer has done the same thing. Big ads on TV. "Get your light beer." Thirty percent fewer calories.

We are only saying "Isn't it about time the egg industry thinks about something like that instead of spending the money fighting all of the research?" You will be arguing until doomsday on what causes heart attacks.

It seems to me a little research in producing a chicken that produces lower cholesterol eggs would put you in the same category with the other industries.

"We are not fighting research," replied Jerry Bookey, an egg producer, but to date, the egg industry cannot claim that it has tried to do for the cholesterol in eggs what the beer industry has done for the calories in beer. Undoubtedly, lowering the cholesterol content of eggs would be more difficult, but a few experiments do suggest that changes in chickens' diets might lower the cholesterol content of eggs. Conceivably, different breeding techniques might also produce a chicken that lays eggs lower in cholesterol. But the egg industry had insisted on arguing, even though it was obvious that a consensus about fat, cholesterol, and heart disease was developing.

Of course, the egg industry was not the only one to ignore the handwriting on the wall. The beef producers also took a defensive approach to the heart research, fighting it rather than trying to accommodate more of their producers to the cardiologists' advice. The dairy industry, though it had long provided low-fat products, also did not prepare for the day of reckoning by seeking reforms in the farmers' milk pricing system that encourages production of surplus fat. Only the pork producers dealt with the fat problem—and with success. Thanks to new techniques, today's hog has much less fat than its ancestors. But the other industries ignored the example of the pork producers. Perhaps they were hoping that their political power would see them through the most convincing scientific evidence.

12

Nutrition Policy at a Crossroads

It was one of the most bizarre moments in the story of fat and cholesterol. Alan Stone, director of the Senate Select Committee on Nutrition and Human Needs, had just finished discussing the committee's *Dietary Goals* report at a 1977 meeting of the Grocery Manufacturers of America, the food industry's largest lobbying organization. When he offered to answer questions about the committee's nutritional advice, a food industry executive rose to ask him an extraordinary question: did he understand the difference between our form of government and the form of government in the Soviet Union? If the *Dietary Goals* report were not a sign of totalitarianism, then it must have been a bedtime story composed by that annoying threat to everyone's happiness: the National Nanny who is forever reminding us not to smoke, to wear our seatbelts, and to have our blood pressures checked.

Today, the food industry has geared up against government recommendations to eat less fat and cholesterol as if the advice were truly a threat to our entire political system. In 1980, food producers launched an intensive lobbying effort against the government's advice—all sparked by the February 1980 publication of an almost innocuous brochure, *Nutrition and Your Health: Dietary Guidelines for Americans*. The pamphlet, a joint publication of the USDA and HHS, contains rather mild advice to "avoid too much fat, saturated fat, and cholesterol." Over this, the food producers are hysterical.

Within days after the pamphlet was released, the USDA received a letter from Senator Herman Talmadge, chairman of the Senate Agriculture Committee, complaining that the USDA and HHS had not allowed farm groups to participate in formulating the recommendations. Talmadge was not the only member of Congress to complain. By the summer of 1980, the USDA had received letters from seventy-five members of Congress, written on behalf of egg producers. Directors of Agriculture in Missouri, Delaware, Vermont, Maryland, Louisiana, Washington, Ohio, and North Carolina also sent protest letters. The Department of Agriculture in Missouri organized a demonstration to protest the USDA-HHS recommendations. Cattle and egg producers quickly brought the protest rally to the attention of Missouri Senator Thomas Eagleton. Eagleton, facing a tough re-election fight in 1980, was in no condition to ignore farm group pressures.

In June 1980, Eagleton write to Bob Bergland, secretary of the USDA, requesting that the department cease distribution of its *Dietary Guidelines* pamphlet. "It is my strong belief that the Department of Agriculture should review in detail the nutritional advice on which it has put its stamp of approval," wrote Eagleton. "Until such time as this review is completed, I strongly recommend that the department suspend distribution of the pamphlet." Eagleton followed his letter to the USDA with a hearing where he blasted USDA and HHS officials for going too far in advising the public about diet. Eagleton, who chairs the Senate Appropriations Subcommittee that oversees funding of the Department of Agriculture, said he would not specifically try to ban distribution of the pamphlet in the next USDA appropriations bill. Instead, he began pressuring the USDA to tone down the pamphlet even more. The USDA has responded to his

231

demands by promising to italicize a statement in the pamphlet that acknowledges a controversy about diet and heart disease. Eagleton has replied that this is not enough.

In the House of Representatives, Congressman Ike Skelton, also from Missouri, sought more drastic measures. In August 1980, Skelton proposed an amendment to the USDA appropriations bill that would have prohibited the agency from publishing or distributing the pamphlet on dietary guidelines. In addition, the amendment would have banned the USDA from distributing any information about the pamphlet "until such time as there has been a complete review of all conclusions contained in the guidelines and they have been established as fact." The amendment was blocked on a technicality. Three months before the 1980 presidential election, the American Farm Bureau Federation wrote to President Carter, requesting that distribution of the pamphlet be halted until revisions are made. The letter insisted that the government lacks "sufficient scientific research basis to promote definite dietary guidelines, particularly as they affect red meats, milk, and egg production."

Though the farm groups had not yet succeeded in halting distribution of the brochure, pressure from the American Meat Institute, a trade group representing meat processors, did force withdrawal of another USDA publication—a meal-planning guide for directors of school lunch programs. The guide suggested efforts to reduce the fat, salt, and sugar content of school lunches. An appendix included a how-to fact sheet listing foods high in fat, salt, and sugar. The meat industry was furious about the fact sheet—which, of course, revealed that processed meats are often high in fat. Senator Eagleton called for withdrawal of the guide. Senator Talmadge wrote the USDA charging that food industry officials had told him that the guide "contains provisions showing an apparent prejudice against beef, pork, milk, and all processed meats and canned vegetables." The guide has been withdrawn, pending revisions. USDA sources say that the revised version will not include the fact sheet listing foods high in fat.

No doubt about it, the government efforts to inform the public about the hazards of a high-fat diet are in jeopardy. But even if the government is silenced, as it well may be, the food producers, too, will be in jeopardy, for they have still other voices to fear. Not all sources of scientific opinion can be as easily squelched as government agencies.

In August 1980, 104 organizations, including consumer groups, labor unions, and scientific societies, joined forces in criticizing industry efforts to squelch the USDA-HHS brochure on dietary guidelines. "We have too often seen industry lobbyists scurrying through the halls of Congress in order to have laws written to promote their interests," said spokeswoman Ellen Haas of the Community Nutrition Institute, "but we have never before seen requests to Congress to rewrite the laws of science and medicine." The American Dietetic Association (ADA), the nation's professional society of dietitians, responded to a congressional inquiry with support for the USDA-HHS guidelines. "*Nutrition and Your Health: Dietary Guidelines for Americans* is an important document in that it addresses the relationship between food choices and health," said the ADA. "We believe that these guidelines represent a definite step in the right direction in emphasizing the maintenance of health through good nutrition." In so many words, the ADA complained that the advice was too wishy-washy. "We . . . eagerly await quantitative guides for further translation of 'too much fat' . . . into daily eating plans," said the group. On behalf of a physician's society, the American College of Preventive Medicine, Dr. Jerome Cohen declared that withdrawal of the USDA-HHS brochure "would be an egregious disservice to the American public."

The grand alliance of nutritionists, government, and food producers has been shattered. Fifty years ago, the three saw themselves as close allies, all working together for mutual benefit. Today, the goals of nutritionists sometimes sharply contradict the goals of the food producers. One need look no further than the Basic Four—once everyone's favorite nutrition advice—for an example. Food producers are working hard to keep the Basic

Four alive. In supporting the National Consumer Nutrition Information Act, a bill to expand government nutrition education programs, the National Milk Producers Federation admitted concerns about the definition of a "healthful diet." The federation urged that nutrition education programs revolve around the nutrient allowances set for protein, vitamins, and minerals—which are, of course, translated into the Basic Four. Nutritionists, on the other hand, are losing faith in the Basic Four. In 1978, the Society for Nutrition Education, a group of professional nutritionists and nutrition educators, passed a resolution urging that the Basic Four be modified and more relevant alternatives developed. "The time is at hand for development of a new food guide," concluded the society. The American Dietetic Association has also acknowledged shortcomings in the Basic Four. "In the past the guides to good eating and food choices stressed food for health, but the effects of inappropriate food choices for health were not emphasized," said the ADA in 1980.

And so, nutritionists are not as enthused as they once were with the National Dairy Council's materials that still feature the Basic Four as the gospel. In 1979, the Society for Nutrition Education passed a resolution that requires nutrition education materials to discuss the relationship between saturated fat, cholesterol, and heart disease when high-fat foods are mentioned, in order to qualify for the group's endorsement. By this standard, almost nothing produced by the Dairy Council would qualify for an endorsement.

Times have also changed since the country's most famous nutritionist, Dr. Elmer McCollum, toured the country saying, "The dairy industry has made us what we are." McCollum's successor as the nation's most famous nutritionist, Dr. Jean Mayer, has instead charged that the same once-idolized dairy industry interfered with Senate hearings on diet and heart disease. "We have the agricultural resources, the medical knowledge, the technology, and the distribution system to make great strides forward," wrote Mayer on that occasion. "But we will not be able to move until politicians of both parties learn to protect the

234

nutrition and health of the American people against the pressures of special interests." He does not sound like Elmer McCollum.

It is not just the partnership between nutritionists and food producers that seems to have dissolved. In the past decade, both the farmers and the nutritionists have grown disillusioned with their one-time ally, the USDA. In a 1972 article entitled "USDA-Built-In Conflicts," Jean Mayer charged that the USDA's record of putting farm interests in front of public health was so glaring that its consumer protection activities should be transferred to a different agency. Mayer charged the USDA with donating "inappropriate foods" to the poor, elderly, and to school feeding programs—foods high in saturated fat, salt, or calories. "USDA-sponsored programs on nutrition education are even more hampered," he wrote. "The mere mention of the words *saturated fat* or *cholesterol* is prevented by powerful dairy and meat pressure groups to which the department always defers." His conclusion would have seemed out of place in 1920, but not in 1972:

> No one concerned with the continued health and prosperity of the nation wants the two million farmers on whom the bulk of our food production depends to be neglected or to be deprived of a voice in government. But neither is there a reason why 15 million poor, 40 million school children, or 206 million consumers should always be subordinated to a special interest group, important though it may be.

At the USDA, officials pleaded guilty as charged—but said that the agency has reformed. In September 1979, Agriculture Secretary Bob Bergland told an audience, "I'm happy to report that the USDA has joined the twentieth century. When I became Secretary of Agriculture some thirty-three months ago, the department had a long tradition of being more responsive to the production and marketing of food than to the safety, quality, and nutritional content of the foods consumers eat. That is now a dead tradition." The USDA's efforts to update its nutrition education materials and improve school lunches testify to a changing agency. But the dairy farmers, for one, are upset with the USDA for requiring that schools offer low-fat or skim milk in the lunchroom. Some schools have responded by serving only low-fat milk. The dairy farmers have had to seek congressional help to tame the agency once so loyal to them. The Senate has passed a bill that would require schools to make whole milk available.

The farmers interpreted even a few changes that they oppose as evidence that the USDA has turned on them. Norma Jean Moseley, an Iowa pork producer, told *The Washington Post* in 1980 that the two things that bothered her the most about the USDA were its new pamphlet on dietary guidelines and its former assistant secretary, Carol Tucker Foreman, who helped initiate the dietary guidelines and USDA efforts to reduce the levels of the food additive sodium nitrite in pork. The farmers believed that Foreman was not only not for them, but out to get them. "Why put somebody in the USDA who is out to hurt the hog farmer?" Moseley told the newspaper. Another sign of paradise lost.

But Foreman, who endured the ire of farmers accustomed to an agency that did everything their way, did not believe that the friction between nutritionist, food producer, and government had to be. Foreman saw her agency's new position on diet as one providing the food producers with new opportunities—not simply a threat to their profits. She believed that they could prosper by cooperating instead of fighting, as she told an audience in 1979:

> The food industry is on the threshold of a major decision, and it may be the most important decision on this entire issue. The food industry—producers, processors, and re-tailers—can choose to dig in and fire away at the national nanny, do-gooder, blankety-blank Surgeon General and [USDA] Human Nutrition Center, or it can choose to grab the information from the Human Nutrition Center and turn it into a major marketing strategy. The industry has taken

such initiatives in the past. They developed enriched flour and polyunsaturated margarines. They reduced the lard weight of pork, and packed fruit in its own juice—to name just a few. . . . The food processors must make a decision. They can gear up and fight to avoid any change in present products, or they can seize the opportunity to market a whole variety of new foods. Certainly they do not lack the capability.

If the food producers took Foreman's advice, the field of nutrition might experience peaceful days once more. But with George McGovern no longer in the Senate, Secretaries Bergland and Foreman no longer at USDA, and congressmen who fought the USDA-HHS dietary guidelines still remaining on Capitol Hill, only a Pollyanna would predict that a truce is imminent.

Using the Appendixes

Appendix I lists the fat content of common foods, classified by categories (cheeses, vegetables, etc.). A listing of the categories precedes the tables. Appendix II covers brand-name foods, by category also. Within each category of this appendix, foods are subdivided by manufacturer. A listing of the categories for Appendix II appears before the second set of tables.

The listings give first, the fat content as a percentage of calories in the food. This value will not change, regardless of serving size. The serving size is included for using the grams-per-serving and calories column. For common foods, the serving sizes have been designated by the U.S. Department of Agriculture. The serving sizes for meat represent cooked portions of choice grade (and remember that 3 ounces, the standard serving size for meat, is a very small portion, as described with the scoreboard in Chapter 7). For the brand-name section, the serving size chosen by the manufacturer was used. For a given item, one manufacturer may assume a different serving size than another. If this is the case, use the percentage-of-calories column to compare among brands. The percentage method will show if there are big differences in fat content when servings sizes are not equal.

Using the Appendixes

The numbers in these tables represent average values found when sampling the fat content of a product. It is normal for fat content of a food to vary somewhat from one piece or one batch to another. Also, please realize that food manufacturers change their recipes from time to time. Therefore, the numbers in these tables can become outdated. For the most up-to-date information, check with the manufacturer.

Listing of a food in these tables does not constitute an endorsement. Some of these foods, even if low in fat, contain large amounts of salt, sugar, or poorly tested food additives. The charts are for your information only.

Due to space limitations, all foods could not be included. For nutrition information on a food not listed, write to the manufacturer. For more information—fat, vitamins, minerals, etc.—in common foods, consult *Handbook 456* of the U.S. Department of Agriculture. A copy of *Handbook 456* can be obtained by sending a check for $5.15 to the Superintendent of Documents, Government Printing Office, Washington, D.C. 20402. Ask for stock number 0100-03184.

Appendix I

FAT CONTENT OF COMMON FOODS

1. Beans, Nuts, and Seeds
2. Beef
3. Breads, Rolls, and Baked Goods
4. Candy
5. Cereals, Grains, and Pasta
6. Dairy Products and Eggs
7. Fish
8. Fruits
9. Lamb
10. Pork
11. Poultry
12. Processed Meats
13. Veal
14. Vegetables

240

Beans, Nuts, and Seeds

		% cal/ fat	Grams fat per serving	Calories per serving
1 cup	Soybeans, cooked	37	10	234
1 piece	Soybeans, curd (tofu), 2½ × 2¾ × 1″	49	5	86
¼ cup	Peanuts, roasted	70	18	210
¼ cup	Sunflower seeds, hulled	71	17	203
2 Tbsp.	Peanut butter	73	16	188
¼ cup	Almonds, roasted	77	23	246
¼ cup	Walnuts, black, chopped, shelled	79	18	196

Less than 20% calories from fat: Beans (all types except soybeans), bean sprouts, chestnuts, chickpeas.

Beef

		% cal/ fat	Grams fat per serving	Calories per serving
3 oz.	Beef liver, raw	25	4	150
3 oz.	Round steak, lean only	29	5	161
3 oz.	Sirloin steak, wedge or roundbone, lean only	33	6	176
3 oz.	Flank steak, 100% lean	33	6	167
1 cup	Stewing beef, lean only	40	13	300
3 oz.	Rump roast, lean only	40	8	177
3 oz.	Beef liver, fried	41	9	195
3 oz.	Porterhouse steak, lean only	42	9	190
3 oz.	T-bone steak, lean only	42	9	190
3 oz.	Sirloin steak, hipbone, lean only	47	11	204
3 oz.	Chuck rib roast or steak, lean only	50	12	212
3 oz.	Rib roast, lean only	50	11	205
3 oz.	Round steak, lean w/ fat	53	13	222

		% cal/ fat	Grams fat per serving	Calories per serving
3 oz.	Ground beef, fairly lean	64	17	235
1 cup	Stewing beef, lean w/ fat	66	34	458
3 oz.	Rump roast, lean w/fat	71	23	295
3 oz.	Sirloin steak, wedge or roundbone, lean w/fat	75	27	329
3 oz.	Chuck rib roast or steak, lean w/fat	78	31	363
3 oz.	Rib roast, lean w/fat	81	34	374
3 oz.	Porterhouse steak, lean w/fat	82	36	395
3 oz.	T-bone steak, lean w/ fat	82	37	402
3 oz.	Sirloin steak, hipbone, lean w/fat	83	38	414

Breads, Rolls, and Baked Goods

	% cal/ fat	Grams fat per serving	Calories per serving
1 med. Doughnut	42	8	164
⅛ commercial ring Danish pastry	49	10	179

Less than 20% of calories from fat: Breads (cracked wheat, French, Italian, white, rye, whole wheat); rolls (frankfurter, Parker House, hard); angel food cake; fig bars; ginger snaps; lady fingers; raisin cookies (biscuit type); animal crackers; pretzels; zweiback.

Candy

		% cal/ fat	Grams fat per serving	Calories per serving
1 oz.	Chocolate, plain	53	9	147

Less than 20% calories from fat: butterscotch, plain mints, gumdrops, marshmallows.

242

Cereals, Grains, and Pasta

		% cal/ fat	Grams fat per serving	Calories per serving
1 Tbsp.	Wheat germ, plain	25	1	23

Note: Granolas contain significant amounts of fat. See brand-name appendix under cereal heading.

Less than 20% of calories from fat: barley, bulgur, macaroni, noodles, oatmeal, rice, spaghetti.

Dairy Products and Eggs

		% cal/ fat	Grams fat per serving	Calories per serving
4 oz.	Ice milk, 5.1% fat by weight	29	4	133
1 cup	Milk, 2% w/nonfat solids	30	5	145
8 oz.	Yogurt, low-fat, plain	21	4	144
½ cup	Cheese, cottage	35	4	112
1 cup	Milk, whole	47	8	159
8 oz.	Yogurt, whole milk, plain	48	8	140
4 oz.	Ice cream, reg. (10% fat by weight)	48	7	127
1 oz.	Cheese, mozzarella, part-skim type	55	5	72
½ cup	Cheese, ricotta, part-skim type	50	10	171
1 lg.	Eggs	64	6	82
4 oz.	Ice cream, rich (16% fat by weight)	64	12	165
1 oz.	Cheese, Swiss	66	8	105
½ cup	Cheese, ricotta, whole-milk type	66	16	216
1 oz.	Cheese, Cheddar	71	9	113
1 oz.	Cheese, brick	72	9	105
1 oz.	Cheese, Camembert	72	7	85

1 oz.	Cheese, blue or Roquefort	73	9	105
1 Tbsp.	Cream, Half & Half	79	2	20
1 lg.	Egg, yolk	79	5	59
1 Tbsp.	Cream, coffee or light	85	3	32
1 Tbsp.	Cream cheese	90	5	52
1 Tbsp.	Cream, light whipping	92	5	45
1 pat	Butter	100	4	36
1 Tbsp.	Butter	100	12	102

About cheeses: the only hard cheeses with a moderate fat content are the part-skim types. All of the following cheeses are made from whole milk and contain 8 to 9 grams of fat per ounce serving (and at least 60% of the calories from fat): blue, brick, brie, caraway, Cheddar, Edam, Gouda, Gruyère, Limburger, Monterey, Muenster, Port du salut, Provolone, Romano, Roquefort, Swiss; and pasteurized processed American, pimento or Swiss.

Less than 20% calories from fat: Buttermilk (made from skim milk), uncreamed cottage cheese, skim milk, sherbert, low-fat cottage cheese, uncreamed farmer cheese.

Fish

		% cal/ fat	Grams fat per serving	Calories per serving
1 cup	Oysters, raw, meat only	25	4	158
3 oz.	Tuna, chunk, oil-packed, drained very well	37	7	169
3 oz.	Salmon, pink	38	5	120
3 oz.	Salmon, smoked	48	8	150
3 oz.	Salmon, sockeye (red)	49	8	146
3 oz.	Sardines, Atlantic, in oil, 1 can drained	49	9	173
3 oz.	Mackerel, Pacific, canned	50	8	153
5 fillets	Anchovies	54	2	135

3 oz.	Herring, Pacific	59	12	177
3 oz.	Tuna, chunk, oil- packed, undrained	63	17	245

Less than 20% of calories from fat: cod, crab, flounder, haddock, halibut, lobster, perch, pollock, scallops, sole, shrimp, light tuna in water, some types of albacore tuna in water.

Fruits

		% cal/ fat	Grams fat per serving	Calories per serving
½ cup	Coconut, shredded	85	14	138
2 × 2 × ½" piece	Coconut, fresh	85	16	156

Less than 20% calories from fat: apples, apple butter, apple juice and sauce, apricots, bananas, blackberries, blueberries, boysenberries, sweet cherries, cranberries, cranberry juice cocktail, dates, figs, grapefruits, lemons, lemonade, lychees, mangos, honeydew melons, nectarines, oranges, papayas, peaches, pears, pineapples, plantains, plums, prunes, raisins, raspberries, strawberries, tangerines, watermelons.

Lamb

		% cal/ fat	Grams fat per serving	Calories per serving
3 oz.	Leg, lean only	34	6	158
3 oz.	Rib chops, lean only	45	9	180
3 oz.	Leg, lean w/fat	61	16	237
3 oz.	Rib chops, lean w/fat	79	31	355

Pork

		% cal/ fat	Grams fat per serving	Calories per serving
3 oz.	Ham, lean only	43	8	159
3 oz.	Boston butt (shoulder), lean only	53	12	207
3 oz.	Ham, lean w/fat	69	19	246
3 oz.	Boston butt (shoulder), lean w/fat	73	24	300
3 oz.	Spareribs	80	33	377
2 med. slices	Bacon	82	8	86

Poultry

		% cal/ fat	Grams fat per serving	Calories per serving
Chicken				
3 oz.	Light meat, w/o skin	23	4	147
3 oz.	Dark meat, w/o skin	43	8	174
3 oz.	Light meat w/skin, roasted	44	9	188
3 oz.	Light meat w/skin, flour-coated and fried	44	10	209
3 oz.	Light meat w/skin, batter-dipped and fried	50	13	235
3 oz.	Dark meat w/skin, flour-coated and fried	53	14	242
3 oz.	Dark meat w/skin, roasted	56	13	21⁵
3 oz.	Dark meat w/skin, batter-dipped and fried	56	16	25³
Turkey				
3 oz.	Light meat w/o skin	18	3	133
3 oz.	Dark meat w/o skin	35	6	159
3 oz.	Light meat w/skin	38	7	167
3 oz.	Dark meat w/skin	47	10	188

Other

3 oz.	Goose meat only	48	11	202
3 oz.	Goose meat w/skin	65	19	259
3 oz.	Duck meat only	50	10	171
3 oz.	Duck meat w/skin	76	24	286

Processed Meats

		% cal/ fat	Grams fat per serving	Calories per serving
2 oz.	Scrapple	58	8	122
2 oz.	Liverwurst	75	14	174
2 oz.	Salami	76	22	256
2 oz.	Frankfurter	80	16	176
2 slices	Bologna	81	7	80
2 oz.	Country-style sausage	81	18	196
2 oz. (2 links)	Pork sausage	83	11	124

Veal

		% cal/ fat	Grams fat per serving	Calories per serving
3 oz.	Round roasts and leg cutlets, lean w/fat	46	9	184
3 oz.	Rib roast, lean w/fat	57	14	229
3 oz.	Breast, lean w/fat	63	18	257

Vegetables

		% cal/ fat	Grams fat per serving	Calories per serving
10 med.	French-fried potatoes, 2–3 ½″ long	43	7	137
1 cup	Hash brown potatoes— from frozen	45	18	347
10 chips	Potato chips	62	8	114
½	Avocado	82	19	188
10 small	Olives, green	91	4	33

Less than 20% calories from fat: asparagus, barley, beets, broccoli, bulgur, Chinese cabbage, carrots, cauliflower, collards, corn, raw garden cress, cucumbers, eggplant, endive, farina, horseradish, kale, kohlrabi, lettuce, mushrooms, mustard greens, okra, onion, parsley, parsnips, peas, sweet pepper, dill pickles, pimentos, potatoes, pumpkins, radish, rutabagas, sauerkraut, spinach, squash, tomatoes, tomato juice, turnips, turnip greens, mixed vegetables, watercress.

Appendix II

FAT CONTENT OF BRAND NAME FOODS

1. Beans and Chili
2. Bread
3. Cake Mixes
4. Cakes, Prepared
5. Candy
6. Canned Meat Products
7. Cereals
8. Cookies
9. Crackers
10. Dressings
11. Frosting Mixes
12. Frozen Dinners
13. Muffins, Rolls & Buns
14. Pancake Mixes
15. Pies, Prepared
16. Pizzas
17. Potatoes

18. Puddings
19. Seafood
20. Snack Foods
21. Soups
22. Spaghetti and Pastas
23. Vegetables

Beans and Chili

		% cal/ fat	Grams fat per serving	Calories per serving
Luck's				
8.5 oz.	Great Northern beans seasoned w/pork	24	7	260
8.5 oz.	Blackeye peas seasoned w/pork	28	8	260
8.5 oz.	Pinto beans seasoned w/pork	29	9	280
Campbell's				
8 oz.	Beans and franks in tomato-molasses sauce	39	16	370
Morton House				
8 oz.	Oven-baked beans in tomato sauce	13	4	270
7.5 oz.	Chili w/beans	48	18	340
7.5 oz.	Chili w/o beans	53	20	340
Armour-Dial				
7.75 oz.	Chili w/beans	54	22	370
7.5 oz.	Chili w/o beans	71	34	430
Hormel				
3.5 oz.	Chili w/beans	50	8	151
3.5 oz.	Chili w/o beans	67	12	162
Chef-Boy-Ar-Dee				
7.5 oz.	Beef chili w/beans	46	17	330
7.5 oz.	Beef chili w/o beans	71	29	370

Bread

Most loaf breads by Pepperidge Farm, Arnold, and Wonder contain less than 15% of calories from fat. None contain more than 25% calories from fat.

Cake Mixes (prepared as directed)

		% cal/ fat	Grams fat per serving	Calories per serving
Pillsbury				
¹⁄₁₂ cake	Angel food cake mixes	0	0	140
3″ sq	Gingerbread	19	4	190
2–1½″ sq	Fudge brownie	30	4	120
2–1½″ sq	Walnut brownie	35	5	130
¹⁄₁₂ cake	Pillsbury Plus cake mixes, butter recipe	38	10	240
¹⁄₁₂ cake	Lemon, dark chocolate, devil's food, German chocolate	42	12	260
¹⁄₁₂ cake	Yellow	42	12	260
Betty Crocker				
¹⁄₁₂ cake	Angel food cake	0	0	130
¹⁄₉ cake	Gingerbread	26	6	210
¹⁄₁₂ cake	Layer cake mixes: white, sour-cream white	27	6	200
¹⁄₃₂ pkg	Date bar mix	30	2	60
¹⁄₁₂ cake	Pound cake mix	38	8	190
¹⁄₁₂ cake	Layer cake mixes: banana, yellow, strawberry, orange, lemon, German chocolate, devil's food	43	13	270

		% cal/ fat	Grams fat per serving	Calories per serving
Duncan Hines				
¹⁄₁₂ cake	Angel food	0	0	140
¹⁄₉ cake	Moist & Easy spicy apple rasin	20	4	180
¹⁄₁₂ cake	Layer cake mixes: spice, yellow, or banana supreme	22	5	200
¹⁄₁₂ cake	Layer cake mix: devil's food	27	6	200
¹⁄₉ cake	Moist & Easy golden chocolate chip	28	6	190
¹⁄₁₆ mix	Double-fudge brownie mix	32	5	140
¹⁄₁₂ cake	Layer cake mix: butter recipe, fudge, and golden	43	13	270
Quaker				
¹⁄₈ cake	Aunt Jemima Easy Mix coffee cake	26	5	170
1 oz = 1 cupcake	Flako cupcake mix	30	5	150
General Foods-Jell-O				
¹⁄₈ cake	Cheesecake	40	11	250

Cakes, Prepared

Sara Lee				
¹⁄₈ cake	Banana cake	36	7	175
1	Chocolate cupcakes	41	9	190
¹⁄₈ cake	Strawberry shortcake	43	9	193
1	Cinnamon rolls	38	4	100
¹⁄₁₀ cake	Pound cake	48	7	124
¹⁄₈ cake	Pecan coffeecake	50	9	165
¹⁄₆ cake	Cream cheese cake	50	13	240
¹⁄₁₀ cake	Chocolate pound cake	47	6	122

Pillsbury

2	Cinnamon rolls w/ icing	31	8	230
2	Caramel danish w/nuts	42	14	300

Hostess

1	Sno Balls	25	4	140
1	Chocolate cupcakes	25	5	160
1	Twinkies	26	4	140
1	Brownie (large)	36	10	240
2	Ho Hos	45	12	240
1	Ding Dongs & Big Wheels	53	10	170

Candy

	% cal/ fat	Grams fat per serving	Calories per serving
Hershey's			
1 oz. Hershey-Ets	38	6	142
1 oz. Rally	47	8	145
1 oz. Kit Kat	47	8	143
1 oz. Krackel	49	8	149
1 oz. Reese's peanut butter cups	53	9	153
1 oz. Milk chocolate bar or Kisses	53	9	156
Nestlé's			
1 oz. $100,000 bar	39	6	140
1 oz. Choco'lite bar, crunch or milk chocolate	48	8	150
1 oz. Almond bar	54	9	150

Canned Meat Products

		% cal/ fat	Grams fat per serving	Calories per serving
Morton House				
6.25 oz.	Gravy and sliced tur-key	39	6	140
5 oz.	Barbecue sauce w/beef for sloppy joes	41	11	240
8 oz.	Beef stew	49	13	240
4⅙ oz.	Mushroom gravy and salisbury steak	62	11	160
Armour-Dial				
1.25 oz.	Sliced dried beef	12	0.8	60
8 oz.	Beef stew	51	12	210
7.6 oz.	Sloppy joe beef	55	20	330
7.63 oz.	Corned beef hash	63	28	400
3 oz.	Treet	81	27	300
Hormel				
3.5 oz.	DINTY MOORE veg-etable stew	44	4	76
3.5 oz.	DINTY MOORE beef stew	45	4	86
3.5 oz.	DINTY MOORE corned beef	53	13	229
3.5 oz.	SPAM luncheon meat	77	26	310
Chef-Boy-Ar-Dee				
7.5 oz.	Meat balls in brown gravy	54	18	300
Swift's Premium				
3.6 oz.	Hostess canned ham	39	6	140
3.6 oz.	Canned ham	61	15	220

254

Cereals

All major brand cereals contain less than 20% of calories from fat except as listed below.

		% cal/ fat	Grams fat per serving	Calories per serving
General Foods-Post				
1 oz.	C. W. Post family style (granola)	30	5	140
Heartland Natural Cereal				
1 oz.	Plain, or with raisins	30	4	120
1 oz.	(about ¼ cup) Coconut variety	35	5	130
Kellogg				
1 oz.	Cracklin' Bran	33	4	110
1 oz.	Country Morning	35	5	130
General Mills				
1 oz.	Nature Valley granola w/fruit & nuts	28	4	130
1 oz.	Nature Valley granola (all other flavors)	35	5	130
Quaker				
1 oz.	100% natural cereal w/ apples & cinnamon	37	5	135
1 oz.	100% natural cereal w/ raisins & dates	38	6	134
1 oz.	100% natural cereal	41	6	139

Cookies

	% cal/ fat	Grams fat per serving	Calories per serving
Sunshine			
1 piece Golden fruit biscuits	9	.6	61
1 piece Fig bars	16	.8	45
1 piece Mallopuffs	23	1.6	63
1 piece Gingersnaps	23	.6	24
1 piece Animal crackers	27	.3	10
1 piece Butter-flavored cookies	35	.9	23
1 piece Oatmeal	36	2.3	58
1 piece Vanilla wafers	36	.6	15
1 piece Hydrox	41	2.2	48
1 piece Chip-a-roos (large)	41	2.9	63
1 piece Chocolate fudge sandwich	46	3.7	72
Frito-Lay			
2 oz. Fig bar	16	3.4	189
2 oz. Creme-filled oatmeal cake	40	11.3	257
2 oz. Choc-o-roon coconut patties	48	15.2	286
Nabisco			
2 Raisin fruit biscuits	8	1	110
2 Fig Newtons	16	2	110
4 Old-fashioned gingersnaps	22	3	120
11 Barnum's animal crackers	28	4	130
7 Nilla wafers	28	4	130
5 Brown-edged wafers	32	5	140
6 Butter-flavored cookies	32	5	140
2 Mallomars chocolate cakes	33	4	110
3 Oreo chocolate sandwich cookies	36	6	150
2 Oatmeal cookies	36	6	150
2 Peanut butter sandwich cookies	39	6	140
3 Chips Ahoy chocolate chips	39	7	160
8 Biscos sugar wafers	42	7	150

3 Chocolate grahams	42	8	170
4 Lorna Doone shortbread	45	8	160
2 Mystic mints	48	9	170

Crackers

	% cal/ fat	Grams fat per serving	Calories per serving
Sunshine			
1 piece Soda crackers	23	.5	20
1 piece Cheez-Its	45	.3	6
Frito-Lay			
1 oz. Cheddar Bitz	33	5	129
1.5 oz. Cheese-filled crackers	42	9	203
1.5 oz. Toasted crackers w/peanut butter	50	12	220
1 oz. Bacon Snacks	55	9	150
Nabisco			
4 pieces Zwieback toast	22	3	120
36 Oysterettes (soup & oyster)	22	3	120
10 Premium saltines	22	3	120
4 Graham crackers	22	3	120
6 Arrowroot biscuits	28	4	130
7 Triscuits	32	5	140
9 Butter Thins	35	5	130
16 Wheat Thins	39	6	140
8 Waverly wafers	39	6	140
14 Sociables	39	6	140
9 Ritz crackers	48	8	150
14 Chicken in a Biskit	51	8	140

Dressings

		% cal/ fat	Grams fat per serving	Calories per serving
Best Foods				
all 1 Tbsp.	Hellmann's spin blend salad dressing	80	5	55
	Hellmann's sandwich spread	86	6	60
	Hellmann's tartar sauce	98	8	70
	Hellmann's real mayonnaise	99	11	100
Lipton-Wish Bone				
all 1 Tbsp.	French low-cal	36	1	25
	Russian low-cal	36	1	25
	Russian	45	3	60
	Italian	90	8	80
	Caesar	90	8	80
	Chunky blue cheese	90	8	80
	Deluxe French	90	5	50
	Creamy garlic	90	8	80

Frosting Mixes (prepared as directed)

		% cal/ fat	Grams fat per serving	Calories per serving
Pillsbury				
¹⁄₁₂ cake	Chocolate fudge, double Dutch, lemon caramel, milk chocolate	26	5	170
¹⁄₁₂ cake	Strawberry, vanilla	32	6	170
Betty Crocker				
¹⁄₁₂ package plus ¼ Tbsp. butter	Most flavors	32	6	170

Frozen Dinners

		% cal/ fat	Grams fat per serving	Calories per serving
Green Giant				
all 3.6 oz.	Chicken chow mein w/o noodles (boil-in-bag entree)	9	1	50
	Beef stew (boil-in-bag)	15	1	65
	Chicken and biscuits (oven-baked entree)	26	3	98
	Macaroni and cheese (boil in bag)	36	5	119
	Stuffed green peppers w/beef in creole sauce (boil in bag)	48	5	101
	Breaded veal parmigiana (oven-baked)	49	9	156
	Salisbury steaks w/ tomato sauce (boil-in-bag)	57	9	146
Swanson				
11.5 oz.	Turkey	28	11	360
11.5 oz.	Beef	29	12	370
10.25 oz.	Ham	31	13	380
12.5 oz.	Macaroni and cheese	32	14	390
10.25 oz.	Fish 'n chips	40	20	450
11.5 oz.	Fried chicken	46	29	570
12.25 oz.	Veal parmigiana	47	27	520
11.5 oz.	Salisbury steak	52	29	500
Morton				
11 oz.	Spaghetti and meatballs	20	8	360
11 oz.	Fried chicken	27	14	470
10.75 oz.	Beans and franks	29	17	530
9 oz.	Fish	30	9	270
10 oz.	Ham	35	17	440
8 oz.	Macaroni and cheese	35	11	280
10 oz.	Beef	37	11	270
10.25 oz.	Chicken croquettes	40	18	410
8 oz.	Beef pot pie	45	16	320
9.5 oz.	Beef tenderloin, rib eye and sirloin strip steak	64	58–65	820–920

Muffins, Rolls, and Buns

	% cal/ fat	Grams fat per serving	Calories per serving
Wonder			
1 English muffins	8	1	130
1 Hot dog or hamburger rolls	16	3	160
2 oz. Brown and serve rolls	27	5	170
Pillsbury			
2 Hungry Jack flaky biscuits	45	9	180
2 Crescents	47	10	190
Pepperidge Farm			
1 Club	8	1	120
½ French rolls (large)	10	2	190
1 Hamburger rolls	25	3	110
3 Parker House rolls	25	5	180
3 Old-fashioned	33	4	110
1 Golden Twists	45	6	120
1 Butter Crescents	48	7	130
Sara Lee			
1 Poppyseed or sesame seed rolls	33	2	55
1 Parker House rolls	33	3	73
Arnold (over 15% calories from fat)			
1 Soft sandwich rolls, plain or poppy seed	16	2	110
1 Deli-twist rolls	16	2	110
4 Dinner party tea rolls	19	3	140
1 Dutch egg sandwich buns	21	3	130
2 Dinner rolls	23	3	120
2 Dinner party fingers, rounds or Parker House rolls	25	3	110
1 Soft sandwich rolls, sesame seeds	25	3	110

The following Arnold products have less than 15% of calories from fat:
San Francisco sourdough French rolls; San Francisco variety rolls (hamburger buns, hot dog buns, English muffins); Oroweat muffins (bran'ola, honey-butter, honey-wheat berry, raisin, sourdough).

Pancake Mixes (prepared as directed)

Fat content may be reduced by using skim milk or less shortening than called for in directions.

		% cal/ fat	Grams fat per serving	Calories per serving
General Foods				
3 x 4" pan-cakes	Log Cabin complete mix	13	3	180
	Log Cabin regular or buttermilk	27–30	6–7	180–230
Pillsbury-Hungry Jack				
3 x 4" pan-cakes	Complete buttermilk	8	3	340
	Complete	12	3	220
	Extra-light	30	6	180
	Buttermilk	41	11	240
Betty Crocker				
3 x 4" pan-cakes	Complete buttermilk	13	3	210
	Buttermilk	30	9	270
Quaker-Aunt Jemima				
3 x 4" pan-cakes	Complete buttermilk	11	3	240
	Complete	14	3	200
	Whole wheat	32	9	250
	Original	33	8	220
	Buttermilk	31	11	300

261

Pies (prepared)

		% cal/ fat	Grams fat per serving	Calories per serving
Mrs. Smith's				
all ⅙ pie	Boston cream	34	13	327
	Lemon meringue	35	10	260
	Pumpkin	36	9	240
	Cherry	40	14	312
	Pecan	42	20	430
	Chocolate, light	43	12	250
	Coconut cream	44	11	230
	Strawberry yogurt	45	10	200
	Apple	46	15	295
	Banana, light	49	12	220
Morton				
all ⅙ pie	Pumpkin	30	8	230
	Apple	40	13	290
	Cherry	42	14	300
	Banana cream	51	10	170
	Coconut cream	54	11	190

Pizzas

	% cal/ fat	Grams fat per serving	Calories per serving
Chef-Boy-Ar-Dee (½ pizza)			
6.5 oz. Pepperoni (large)	32	14	390
7.75 oz. Deluxe (large)	33	16	430
7 oz. Hamburger (large)	33	16	440
Armour-Dial (½ pizza)			
6.75 oz. Appian Way cheese	24	12	450

Quaker-Celeste (¼ pizza)

4.75 oz. Cheese	36	13	320
5.875 oz. Deluxe	45	19	367
5 oz. Pepperoni	46	18	356
5.5 oz. Sausage	47	20	375

Potatoes

	% cal/ fat	Grams fat per serving	Calories per serving
General Foods-Birds Eye			
3 oz. Crinkle cut	30	4	110
2.8 oz. Cottage fries	34	5	120
3.2 oz. Tiny Taters	54	12	200
Betty Crocker			
½ cup Potatoes au gratin★	36	6	150
½ cup Scalloped potatoes★	36	6	150

★prepared as directed

Puddings

	% cal/ fat	Grams fat per serving	Calories per serving
Del Monte			
3.6 oz. Vanilla	25	4	130
3.6 oz. Chocolate or butterscotch	26	4	126
General Foods-Jell-O			
½ cup All Jell-O instant puddings and pie fillings			
w/skim milk	less than 15	1	150 (approx.)
w/whole milk (coconut creme somewhat higher)	24	5	180–190

		% cal/ fat	Grams fat per serving	Calories per serving
Hunt-Wesson Foods (snack pack puddings)				
5 oz.	Lemon	26	4	140
5 oz.	Tapioca	35	5	130
5 oz.	Rice	38	8	190
5 oz.	All other flavors	47–52	10–11	180–200

Seafood

		% cal/ fat	Grams fat per serving	Calories per serving
Del Monte				
3.6 oz.	Bonito	67	19	257
Mrs. Paul's				
3 oz.	(4) Fish sticks	30	5	150
4 oz.	(2) Fish cakes	34	8	210
3.5 oz.	Fried scallops	34	8	210
4 oz.	(2) Fried haddock fillets	35	9	230
4 oz.	(2) Fried fish fillets	37	9	220
3 oz.	(1) Deviled crabs	39	7	160
5 oz.	Fish au gratin	43	12	250
4.25 oz.	Flounder w/lemon butter	48	8	150
2.5 oz.	Fried clams	53	16	270
5.5 oz.	Clam crepes	55	17	280
3 oz.	Fried shrimp	58	11	170
5 oz.	(2) Buttered fish fillets	75	26	310

Snack Foods

		% cal/ fat	Grams fat per serving	Calories per serving
Frito-Lay				
1 ⅜ oz.	Toasted corn nuggets	28	5	176
1 oz.	Doritos tortilla chips	42	6	137
1 oz.	Cheetos cheese-flavored snacks, puffed	58	10	160
1 oz.	Fritos corn chips	59	10	156
1 oz.	Lay's potato chips	61	10	158
Nabisco				
1 oz.	26 Cheese Nips	42	7	150
Proctor & Gamble				
1 oz.	Pringle's potato chips	60	10	150
Borden				
1 oz.	Cracker Jack	23	3	120

Soups

		% cal/ fat	Grams fat per serving	Calories per serving
Progresso				
all 8 oz.	Tomato	8	1	110
	Clam chowder	9	1	100
	Lentil	13	18	150
	Chickarina	45	5	100
Campbell's (prep. = prepared)				
10 prep. oz.	Tomato	16	2	110
10 prep. oz.	Vegetable	18	2	100
10.75 un-diluted oz.	Chunky vegetable	24	4	150

		% cal/ fat	Grams fat per serving	Calories per serving
10 prep. oz.	Minestrone	25	3	110
10 prep. oz.	Clam chowder (Manhattan or New England)	27	3	100
10 prep. oz.	Beef noodle or chicken noodle	30	3	90
10.75 un- diluted oz.	Chunky chicken	31	8	230
10.75 un- dilted oz.	Chunky beef	33	8	220
10 prep. oz.	Chicken vegetable	40	4	90
10 prep. oz.	Cream of chicken	58	9	140
10 prep. oz.	Cream of mushroom	66	11	150

Lipton

6 oz.	Green pea Cup-a-Soup	8	1	120
6 oz.	Tomato Cup-a-Soup	13	1	70
8 oz.	Green pea soup	14	2	130
8 oz.	Vegetable beef soup	15	1	60
6 oz.	Vegetable beef Cup-a- Soup	15	1	60
8 oz.	Beef mushroom soup	20	1	45
6 oz.	Chicken noodle w/meat Cup-a-Soup	20	1	45
8 oz.	Chicken noodle w/ chicken meat noodle soup	26	2	70
6 oz.	Onion Cup-a-Soup	30	1	30
6 oz.	Cream of chicken Cup- a-Soup	34	3	80
6 oz.	Cream of mushroom Cup-a-Soup	34	3	80

Spaghetti and Pastas

		% cal/ fat	Grams fat per serving	Calories per serving
Chef Boy-Ar-Dee				
7.5 oz.	Cheese ravioli in tomato sauce	20	5	220
7.5 oz.	Beef ravioli in sauce	21	5	210
5.88 oz.	Spaghetti and meatballs dinner	25	9	320
6 oz.	Lasagna dinner	26	9	310
8 oz.	Beefaroni	31	9	260
8 oz.	Spaghetti and meatballs w/tomato sauce	31	8	230
8 oz.	Lasagna	32	10	280
7.5 oz.	Spaghetti w/ground beef in tomato sauce	39	9	210
Campbell's				
7.5 oz.	Beef ravioli in meat sauce	16	4	220
7.25 oz.	Spaghetti w/meatballs in tomato sauce	39	9	210

Vegetables

		% cal/ fat	Grams fat per serving	Calories per serving
General Foods-Birds Eye				
3.3 oz.	Carrots w/brown sugar glaze	23	2	80
3 oz.	French green beans w/ almonds	43	2	50
2.6 oz.	Mixed vegetables w/ onion sauce	47	5	100
3 oz.	Creamed spinach	50	4	60
2.6 oz.	Peas w/cream sauce	51	7	120
3.3 oz.	Broccoli w/hollandaise	72	9	100

Green Giant				
all 3.5 oz.	Golden corn in butter sauce (niblets)	25	3	93
	Boil-in-bag Chinese-style vegetables	30	2	48
	Le Sueur tiny peas, onions & carrots in butter sauce	35	3	71
	Broccoli, cauliflower & carrots in cheese sauce	36	2	55
	Creamed spinach	39	3	74
	Carrots in butter sauce	42	2	49
	Asparagus in butter sauce	56	3	48
Mrs. Paul's				
2.5 oz.	Fried onion rings	42	7	150
4 oz. (2)	Apple fritters	45	12	240
5.5 oz.	Eggplant parmesan	58	16	250

Further Readings*

Atherosclerosis
Cancer
Fat Content of Foods and Our Diet
Government Nutrition Policy
The Government's Nutrition Recommendations
Hearings, U.S. House of Representatives
Hearings, U.S. Senate
History of Nutrition

Atherosclerosis

Ferguson, J. M., and Taylor, C. B. *A Change for Heart,* Palo Alto, CA, Bull Publishing, 1978. A step-by-step guide to eating less saturated fat, cholesterol, salt, and sugar. To order by mail send $4.95 to Bull Publishing, P.O. Box 208, Palo Alto, California 94302.

*A complete list of references used in *Jack Sprat's Legacy* is available from the Center for Science in the Public Interest. Please send $1.50 to cover printing and postage to CSPI-References, 1755 S Street, N.W., Washington, D.C. 20009.

McGill, H. (ed.). *The Geographic Pathology of Atherosclerosis.* Baltimore, Williams and Wilkins, 1968. This book contains all the findings of the International Atherosclerosis Project.

Keys, A. (ed.). Coronary heart disease in seven countries. *Circulation 41:* Supplement 1, 1970. The "Seven Countries" study is a classic one that stands out for its painstaking measurements of the fat content of the subjects' diets.

Stamler, J. Lifestyles, major risk factors, proof, and public policy. *Circulation 58:* 3, 1978. This paper is an excellent summary of the many kinds of evidence linking diet and heart disease.

Conference on the health effects of blood lipids. *Preventive Medicine 8:* 1, 1979. The entire issue of this journal is devoted to interesting and thorough summaries of the many kinds of evidence linking diet and heart disease.

Symposium: The evidence relating six dietary factors to the nation's health. *American Journal of Clinical Nutrition 32:* 2621, 1979. This report discusses the risks and benefits of diets lower in fat and cholesterol.

Wissler, R. W., and Vesselinovitch, D. Experimental models of human atherosclerosis. *Annals of the New York Academy of Sciences 149:* 907, 1968.

Wissler, R. W.. and Vesselinovitch, D. Studies of regression of advanced atherosclerosis in experimental animals and man. *Annals of the New York Academy of Sciences 275:* 363, 1976.

Keys, A., Anderson, J. T., and Grande, F. Serum cholesterol response to changes in the diet. II. The effect of cholesterol in the diet. *Metabolism 14:* 759, 1965.

Keys, A., Anderson, J. T., and Grande, F. Serum cholesterol responses to changes in the diet. IV. Particular saturated fatty acids. *Metabolism 14:* 776, 1965.

Hegsted, D. M., *et al.* Quantitative effects of dietary fat on serum cholesterol in man. *American Journal of Clinical Nutrition 17:* 281, 1965.

Mahley, R. W., *et al.* Alterations in human high-density lipoproteins, with or without increases in plasma cholesterol, induced by diets high in cholesterol. *Lancet 2:* 807, 1978. This study

270

suggests that dietary cholesterol may have adverse effects on HDL-cholesterol levels.

Kannel, W. B., *et al.* Serum cholesterol, lipoproteins, and the risk of coronary heart disease. The Framingham Study. *Annals of Internal Medicine 74:* 1, 1971.

Castelli, W. P., *et al.* HDL-cholesterol and other lipids in coronary heart disease. The cooperative lipoprotein phenotyping study. *Circulation 55:* 767, 1977.

Robertson, T. L., *et al.* Epidemiologic studies of coronary heart disease and stroke in Japanese men living in Japan, Hawaii, and California. *American Journal of Cardiology 39:* 244, 1977. This study and the next one support the concept that smoking and high blood pressure greatly increase the risk of heart disease only when blood cholesterol levels are typically high.

Miettinen, M., *et al.* Effect of cholesterol-lowering diet on mortality from coronary heart disease and other causes. *Lancet 2:* 835, 1972.

Rosen, S., Olin, P., and Rosen, H. V. Dietary prevention of hearing loss. *Acta Otolaryngology 70:* 242, 1970.

Spencer, J. T. Hyperlipoproteinemias in the etiology of inner ear disease. *The Laryngoscope 83:* 639, 1973.

Renaud, S., and Nordoy, A. (eds.). *Dietary Fats and Thrombosis.* Basel, Karger, 1974. This book contains studies on the effect of fat on blood clotting.

Froelicher, V. F., and Oberman, A. Analysis of epidemiologic studies of physical inactivity as risk factor for coronary artery disease. *Progress in Cardiovascular Diseases 15:* 41, 1972.

Federation of American Societies for Experimental Biology. *Evaluation of the Health Aspects of Hydrogenated Soybean Oil as a Food Ingredient.* Springfield, Virginia. National Technical Information Service, 1976. This report evaluates "trans" fats found in margarines and shortenings. For a copy send $4 to the NTIS, U.S. Department of Commerce, Springfield, Virginia 22161. Ask for this publication by its title, but also add its publication number: PB 266 280.

Gordon, T., *et al.* Differences in coronary heart disease in

Framingham, Honolulu, and Puerto Rico. *Journal of Chronic Diseases 27:* 329, 1974.

Chobanian, A. V., *et al.* Body cholesterol metabolism in man. I. The equilibration of serum and tissue cholesterol. *Journal of Clinical Investigation 41:* 1732, 1962. This is a fascinating study that shows cholesterol in the blood migrating into arterial plaques.

Dayton, S., *et al.* A controlled clinic trial of a diet high in unsaturated fat. *Circulation 39, 40:* Suppl. 2, 1969. This report contains findings of the Los Angeles Veterans Study.

Cancer

Tannenbaum, A. The genesis and growth of tumors. III. Effects of a high-fat diet. *Cancer Research 2:* 468, 1942. This was the first experiment showing that fat promotes breast cancer in animals.

Nutrition in the Causation of Cancer. *Cancer Research 35:* 3231, 1975. This entire issue is devoted to diet and cancer. Section II is particularly good.

Carroll, K. K., and Khor, H. T. Dietary fat in relation to tumor genesis. *Progress in Biochemical Pharmacology 10:* 308, 1975. This paper is an outstanding summary of the animal and epidemiological research linking certain cancers to fat intake.

Armstrong, B., and Doll, R. Environmental factors and cancer incidence and mortality in different countries. *International Journal of Cancer 15:* 617, 1975.

Weisburger, J. Colon Cancer: its epidemiology and experimental production. *Cancer 40:* 2414, 1977. This paper is a good update on recent research.

Liu, K., *et al.* Dietary cholesterol, fat, and fiber, and colon-cancer mortality. *Lancet 2:* 782, 1979.

Cruse, J. P., *et al.* Dietary fiber, vivonex, cholesterol and experimental colon cancer. *Gut 19:* A983, 1978.

Haenszel, W., and Kurihara, M. Studies of Japanese migrants. I. Mortality from cancer and other diseases among Japanese in the United States. *Journal of the National Cancer Institute 40:* 43,

1968. This is the major study documenting changes in cancer patterns among Japanese immigrants.

Carroll, K. K., and Hopkins, G. J. Dietary polyunsaturated fat versus saturated fat in relation to mammary carcinogenesis. *Lipids 14:* 155, 1979. This is an important study that may explain why polyunsaturated fat sometimes causes more tumors in animals while human epidemiological studies implicate all fats.

Ederer, F., *et al.* Cancer among men on cholesterol-lowering diets. *Lancet 2:* 203, 1971. This paper combines results of five experiments and shows no excess cancer among men consuming diets high in polyunsaturated fat.

Pearce, M. L., and Dayton, S. Incidence of cancer in men on a diet high in polyunsaturated fat. This is the study which found an excess of cancer deaths among men assigned to a diet high in polyunsaturates.

Hill, M. J. The effect of some factors on the fecal concentration of acid steroids, neutral steroids, and urobilins. *Journal of Pathology 104:* 239, 1971. This study shows how diet affects bile acids.

Reddy, B. S., and Wynder, E. L. Large bowel carcinogenesis: Fecal constituents of populations with diverse incidence rates of colon cancer. *Journal of the National Cancer Institute 50:* 1437, 1973. This survey shows that bile acid excretion varies dramatically among different populations.

Hill, P., and Wynder, E. L. Diet and prolactin release. *Lancet 2:* 806, 1976.

Hill, P., *et al.* Diet, life-style, and menstrual activity. *American Journal of Clinical Nutrition 33:* 1192, 1980. This experiment documents changes in hormone patterns when the fat content of women's diets was increased.

Fat Content of Foods and Our Diet

Carroll, M. D., and Abraham, S. Fats, cholesterol, and sodium intake in the diet of persons 1–74 years. *Advance Data,* No. 54,

1979. This newsletter is available from the National Center for Health Statistics, Hyattsville, Maryland 20782.

Page, L., and Friend, B. The changing United States diet. *Bioscience 28:* 192, 1978. An article discussing how the American diet has changed during the twentieth century.

Adams, C. *Nutritive Value of American Foods* (Agriculture Handbook 456), Washington, D.C. U.S. Department of Agriculture, 1975. The values in this handbook are based on analyses done in the early 1960s. USDA is currently updating its figures. The new handbooks are far more thorough and USDA is issuing them in sections. At this writing the following were available: Handbook 8-1 (dairy and egg products); 8-2 (spices); 8-3 (baby foods); 8-4 (fats and oils); and 8-6 (soups and sauces). All of these handbooks are available from the Government Printing Office, Washington, D.C. 20402. Make checks payable to Superintendent of Documents. Stock Nos. and prices are as follows:

Handbook 456	0100–03184	$5.15
Handbook 8-1	001–000–03635–1	$3.00
Handbook 8-2	001–000–03646–7	$1.30
Handbook 8-3	001–000–03900–8	$5.00
Handbook 8-4	001–000–03984–9	$4.75
Handbook 8-6	001–000–04114–2	$7.00

Government Nutrition Policy

Christopher, T. W., and Dunn, C. W. *Special Federal Food and Drug Laws: Statutes, Regulations, Legislative History, and Annotations.* Chicago, Commerce Clearinghouse, 1954. This is a valuable reference work that should be available in a law school library. Chapter 7 covers the Filled Milk Act, revealing that science once considered milk fat essential to health.

Murphy, E., Page, L., and Koons, P. Lipid Components of Type A School Lunches. *Journal of the American Dietetic Association 56:* 504, 1970. This study found that school lunches contain more saturated fat than the average American diet.

Further Readings

Federal and State Standards for the Composition of Milk Products.
Washington, D.C. U. S. Department of Agriculture, 1977.
This pamphlet gives state standards for almost all dairy
products. It is updated every three years. The 1977 version was
used in this book, but the 1980 update will be available by
winter 1981. Free copies are available from USDA, Washington, D. C. 20250. Ask for Agriculture Handbook # 51.

Mayer, J. (ed.). In: *U.S. Nutrition Policies in the Seventies.* San
Francisco, Freeman and Company, 1973. This book contains a
variety of articles about nutrition policy. "USDA: Built-In
Conflicts" is a particularly good essay about the difficulties in
serving both the public and the food producers at the same
time.

The Government's Nutrition Recommendations

U.S. Senate, Select Committee on Nutrition and Human Needs,
Dietary Goals for the United States. Second Edition, 1977
(December). Available from Government Printing Office,
Washington, D.C. 20402. Include check for $2.30 payable to
Superintendent of Documents and request Stock No.
052–070–04376–8.

*Healthy People: The Surgeon General's Report on Health Promotion
and Disease Prevention.* Washington, D. C. U. S. Dep't of
Health, Education and Welfare, 1979. Available from Government Printing Office, Washington, D.C. 20402. Include check
for $5.00 payable to Superintendent of Documents and request
Stock No. 017–001–00416–2.

Statement on Diet, Nutrition and Cancer. Bethesda, National Cancer
Institute, 1979. Available at no charge from the Office of
Cancer Communications, National Cancer Institute, Bethesda,
Maryland 20205.

Dietary Guidelines for Americans. Washington, D.C. U.S. Depart-
ment of Agriculture and Health and Human Services, 1980.
Available free of charge from Office of Governmental and
Public Affairs, Publication Division, USDA, Washington,
D.C. 20250.

Hearings, U.S. House of Representatives

Note: Free copies of these hearing records may be available from the Nutrition Subcommittee, House Agriculture Committee, 1301 Longworth Bldg., Washington, D.C. 20515. Once out of print, copies can often be found in large libraries.

U.S. House of Representatives. Committee on Agriculture. Hearing: Nutrition Education. September 27–28, 1977. A review of USDA's nutrition information materials begins on page 297.

U.S. House of Representatives. Committee on Agriculture. Hearing: Nutrition Education: National Consumer Nutrition Information Act. January 31, April 12 and 18, June 27, 1978. This hearing record includes the positions of various organizations and industries on a bill that would have expanded government nutrition education programs.

Hearings, U.S. Senate

Note: Congressional committees have a limited supply of their hearing records and will send them free of charge while the supply lasts. Requests should be addressed to the individual committee, U.S. Senate, Washington, D.C. 20510. However, most hearing records of the Senate Select Committee on Nutrition and Human Needs are out of print, and the few that remain can be obtained only through the Government Printing Office, Washington, D.C. 20402. There is a charge for these records, as listed below. Well-stocked libraries often have hearing records.

U.S. Senate. Select Committee on Nutrition and Human Needs. Hearing: Diet Related to Killer Diseases, Volume I. Diet and Cancer. July 27 and 28, 1976 (out of print).

U.S. Senate. Select Committee on Nutrition and Human Needs. Hearing: Diet Related to Killer Diseases, Volume II, Part I. Cardiovascular Disease, February 1 and 2, 1976 (out of print).

A thorough volume filled with easy-to-read information about diet and heart diseases.

U.S. Senate. Select Committee on Nutrition and Human Needs. Diet Related to Killer Diseases, Volume III. Response: Re Meat. March 24, 1977. At this hearing, the meat industry presented its case against the *Dietary Goals for the United States*. Available from Government Printing Office, $4.00. Request Stock No. 052–070–04256–1. See ordering information above.

U.S. Senate. Select Committee on Nutrition and Human Needs. Hearing: Diet Related to Killer Diseases, VI, Response: Re Eggs. July 26, 1977. At this hearing, the egg industry presented its arguments against the *Dietary Goals for the United States* (out of print).

U.S. Senate. Select Committee on Nutrition and Human Needs. Hearing: Nutrition and Human Needs, Part 13-B. July 22–25, 1969. The story of FDA's resistance to fat labeling begins on page 4285 of this hearing (out of print).

U.S. Senate. Committee on Agriculture, Nutrition and Forestry. Hearing: Nutrition and Cancer Research. June 12 and 13, 1978. This hearing focused on the inadequacies of the National Cancer Institute's nutrition research program.

U.S. Senate. Committee on Agriculture, Nutrition and Forestry. Hearing: Heart Disease: Public Enemy No. 1. May 22, 1979. At this hearing, the National Cancer Institute presented its diet recommendations for the public.

History of Nutrition

McCollum, E. V. *From Kansas Farm Boy to Scientist: The Autobiography of Elmer Verner McCollum*. Lawrence, University of Kansas Press, 1964. This book may be ordered by mail from the publisher; include check for $8.31. It's enjoyable reading that will also lend insight into the nutrient orientation that has dominated the science of nutrition.

Hill, M. M., and Cleveland, L. E. Food guides—their development and use. *Nutrition Program News,* July–October 1970. This newsletter gives a history of the Basic Seven and Basic Four. It may be difficult to find in libraries, but is available from the U.S. Department of Agriculture, Consumer Food Economics Institute, Washington, D.C. 20250.

Osborne, T. B., and Mendel, L. B. Amino acids in nutrition and growth. *Journal of Biological Chemistry 17:* 325, 1914. This paper and the next two are classics in protein research.

Osborne, T. B., and Mendel, L. B. The comparative nutritive value of certain proteins in growth and the problem of the protein minimum. *Journal of Biological Chemistry 20:* 351, 1915.

Sumner, E.E., and Murlin, J. R. The biological value of milk and egg protein in human subjects. *Journal of Nutrition 16:* 141, 1938.

Food and Agriculture Organization-World Health Organization. Protein Requirements. WHO Technical Reports Series No. 301, Geneva, World Health Organization, 1965. This report was the basis for using egg as the protein standard.

Committee on Amino Acids-Food and Nutrition Board. *Improvement of Protein Nutriture,* Washington, D.C. National Academy of Sciences, 1974. This recent report concluded that egg should not be the protein standard.

Kuhn, T. S. *The Structure of Scientific Revolutions.* Chicago, University of Chicago Press, 1970. This book is available from the publisher for $3.95. It is a classic book, one that every science student should read. Kuhn bases much of his theory on examples from the physical sciences, but the reaction of nutritionists to evidence challenging their long-held beliefs follows many of the patterns that Kuhn observes in physics and astronomy.

278

Index